THE SECRET FOOTBALLER:
WHAT THE PHYSIO SAW

The Secret Footballer is the author of:

I Am The Secret Footballer
Tales from The Secret Footballer
The Secret Footballer's Guide to the Modern Game
The Secret Footballer: Access All Areas
The Secret Footballer: How to Win
The Secret Footballer: What Goes on Tour

Follow The Secret Footballer on Twitter @TSF

THE SECRET FOOTBALLER

WHAT THE PHYSIO SAW

BANTAM PRESS

LONDON · NEW YORK · TORONTO · SYDNEY · AUCKLAND

TRANSWORLD PUBLISHERS
61–63 Uxbridge Road, London W5 5SA
www.penguin.co.uk

Transworld is part of the Penguin Random House group of companies
whose addresses can be found at global.penguinrandomhouse.com

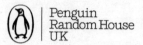

First published in Great Britain in 2018 by Bantam Press
an imprint of Transworld Publishers

A CIP catalogue record for this book
is available from the British Library.

ISBN 9780593078761

Typeset in 11.5/15.25 pt Minion by Jouve (UK), Milton Keynes
Printed and bound in Great Britain by Clays Ltd, Bungay, Suffolk

Penguin Random House is committed to a sustainable
future for our business, our readers and our planet. This book
is made from Forest Stewardship Council® certified paper.

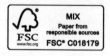

1 3 5 7 9 10 8 6 4 2

To all those who read, heard or saw something from
TSF that changed their opinion of football,
To all those who bought a book, read a column or shared a post,
To all the teammates who looked the other way, passed on
inside stories or shared a changing room, pitch, table,
bar or bed with me,
To all those people in the game who supported me, turned
on me or hanged me,

You have all kept me sane . . .

The Secret Footballer

Contents

Foreword by Mrs TSF

Every football club has a local private hospital that it uses to treat its players. At one particular Premier League club that my husband played for, the hospital made tuna sandwiches for the convalescents. I don't know what they did to those sandwiches but they were amazing. They'd wheel him back into the room and I'd forget he was even there as I watched his TV and ate his sarnies.

When he used to go and see Dr Dodgy Rodge in Leicester it was great because I would get to go to Borders bookshop and read while drinking a latte in the upstairs Starbucks. I love books and I miss Borders. He would come home and say that he had to go to Leicester and I'd say, 'Oh, can I come?'

I never saw the pain. The club hid it from me. The doctors hid it from me. He hid it from me. Even when he was in pain he'd say that he was fine. If he came home hobbling after a match, or maybe on crutches, or with a clutch of pills from the doctor or some stitches in his head, he'd just say, 'Don't worry, it's just a precaution.'

That sounds callous, but he was that way as much for his

own benefit as for mine. They all are. If he told himself that he was fine, that he could carry on, that he wouldn't be out for too long, then it helped his recovery process. He had to play. Footballers have to play. They don't have time to sit and watch somebody take their place, especially when they know that they would be in the first eleven but for the hamstring injury they've suffered.

I can remember him putting his tooth through his lip, breaking his nose, his eyelid hanging off by a thread, having his knees rebuilt, breaking his ribs. And we put a brave face on it. It was football. Theatre. If a guy from any other walk of life came through the door in the state a footballer sometimes does then it would be a major event. But it's just a regular part of the job for us, as it is for every other football couple. Certain aspects of being a footballer lead to players suppressing their emotions, just as much as others lead them to express them – anger in the face of defeat, frustration, or the joy of an unnatural high after beating Huddersfield 1-0.

There were bad injuries of course, and I've often heard him say that he wished he could have his old physio back to help him. That's the problem with moving clubs. Physios have their own way of doing things and if you've been at one club for a long time and you've become used to doing things in a particular way, it can be quite hard to change.

I read something my husband wrote about the fans only seeing footballers for ninety minutes every week and judging them solely on that ninety minutes. There is so much that you don't see, so much that is kept away from the fans and the media. What the physio sees is a big part of football, and what I saw was a combination of physical and mental suffering. TSF once told me that if he had to give an average figure for how physically fit he was throughout his career when he played matches then he would put it at around 80 per cent. Most footballers would probably say the same thing. From the start they are used and abused, then spat out the other end with the body of a sixty-year-old.

That said, I prefer him today. Or maybe I just acknowledge his feelings a little more. He was far too toned when he played football. They all are. There's nothing to grab on to.

Some footballers are like fine wines: they get better with age. My husband's scars add to his personality. But it could be that I just feel sorry for him these days.

Introduction

When mankind learned to stand upright and walk we should have just left it at that. Running was too much. Show-off stuff. Ostentatious. Look at us on our hind legs! Ooh look, we can even go fast without falling over!

For me, running is the single most boring activity known to the species. Bar golf. Running, spending time in the gym and golf are the express routes to insanity.

When I played football I ran around a football pitch because everybody else was doing it and that seemed like the only way of actually getting the ball. There are only a few other circumstances where you might hear the pitter-patter of my perfectly formed feet. If somebody is chasing me with a curved blade and a crazed look (not you, Mrs TSF), well, then I run. So, football and an imminent stabbing – and last orders at a bar a hundred yards away. Outside of those circumstances I have never seen the need for running.

I don't even do the man jog that you see some guys doing when they think their car has been stolen from the supermarket car park. Usually they've just forgotten where they parked.

If I trip over some broken pavement then I gracefully allow my face to hit the concrete rather than disguise the tripping motion by breaking into a light jog, as if I had suddenly been overcome by a spurt of energy.

For those who know me, there was therefore some surprise when on 5 July 2016 (with both English football and the English economy crumbling all around me) I let it be known that the time had come for me to buck the trend and do something radical about my health. I announced my intention to experiment with exercise. My regime would still heavily emphasize the importance of rest but it would now include some running.

I'd had two glorious and happy sedentary years during which I had never even accidentally broken into a jog. Two years where I'd taken a completely hands-off approach to my physique, letting it grow and soften in interesting ways.

The results of this laissez-faire health policy were starting to show. I was never the type of player who was going to 'blow up' once I'd finished football. Those players are cursed with wide diaphragms and broad chests, perfect for bloating through a bad diet once retirement puts an end to all that running about. I had noticed, however, that my lungs appeared to have shrunk and any sort of exertion was causing them to work overtime.

So it's early July, and it's as if my body clock has properly kicked in. The first day of July has always been a historic one in the football calendar: it's when the fun stops and attention turns to pre-season training. I know exactly what all the lads at football clubs up and down the country are doing at this hour of the day. I know the type of running they will be doing and the cruel and unusual punishments they'll inflict on themselves in the afternoon gym session. I think of them fondly and hope that they are vomiting up their intestines.

Remembering the exercises isn't the problem for me: trying to forget them is my trouble. I don't have a team any more, or a master to obey. There is no peer pressure, nobody kicking my arse. I don't have to do anything for anyone. Nobody tells me where I have to be, what time I have to be there, and what I have to do when I arrive. But I get bad flashbacks when sprinting, running up hills, lifting heavy things, even just sweating – endeavours I wasn't designed for.

Football has let go of my hand now, though.

It sounds like the path to paradise, but the Devil rides shotgun with you the whole way. As one of my old sports scientists used to say, 'Anyone can fall down a hole, it's easy; the real difficulty is climbing back out.' I've played for time, forlornly looking at myself in the mirror until realizing that I've landed at the centre of the fucking Earth. That's how big the hole is, and in fairness not everybody can fall down a hole that fucking big. Climbing out is going to take more of an effort than eating fruit for breakfast and running upstairs for a nap.

I've splashed out on some running gear. Or, to give the gear its correct technical name, some leisurewear. In it, I feel better instantly. Maybe I've just been wearing the wrong clothes for feeling fit.

As I head out of the door without my car keys, my wife asks me sweetly if I mightn't like a lift. Then she laughs – more of a cackle, actually. Scary cow.

This business of going for a run is an unnatural act. Nature knows this and conspires against me. June was the wettest June on record, but today, 5 July, has clocked my intentions and decided to make it a scorcher. The great air conditioner in the sky has been switched off. It's muggy out there. Too muggy. Humid. Too humid. Still, a short run through the Amazonian rainforest must be worth at least three long runs through rainy suburbia. If I survive these tropical conditions I give myself permission to take the rest of the week off.

I look up at the blue sky and sample the soupy stillness of the air and my mind dredges up flashbacks of nice days spent sitting by the river watching boats go past. The song 'Drinking in L.A.' slips into my consciousness, because on those nice days I too did nothing. I'm now desperately motivated to go to LA and do some drinking there. I feel the first telltale signs of depression slinking around my brain. Maybe not LA today. Maybe just run to the river and sit for a while. LA will wait.

I instinctively break into the first steps of what I remember to be a jog. I've not even covered a hundred yards when my left hamstring has a panic attack and yanks the emergency cord. My self-preservation department immediately contacts the temporal lobe in my brain to request all available memories pertaining to 'hamstring tears'. It draws a blank. This is a crisis. We are Code Red already. I can't turn back though without having at least run till I'm out of sight of the house.

What we have here is what physiotherapists refer to as a dull ache, rather than a full-on tear which feels as if somebody has stabbed the back of your leg and left the knife in, so that every time you move the blade snags at the flesh. Still, many is the dull ache that has turned into a screaming-in-agony, full-scale, ten-out-of-ten pain. Should I be taking the risk? Maybe I have developed an impossibly high pain threshold and the further my bravery takes me the greater the damage I am doing to myself. I am a tragedy unfurling at a very slow pace.

Rounding the bend from my house and jogging down the hill to the main road reveals that the 'dull ache' is in fact localized, which means it's always in the same place, suggesting that there is in fact some 'trauma'. I'm jogging and I'm suffering trauma. I fucking knew it. Comic Relief has been given enough airtime: Lenny Henry needs to start a telethon for men like me, men who are victims of their own courage. I can see Davina McCall doing a teary-eyed piece to camera as I bravely drag my limping form past her in my leisurewear. That'll light up the phone lines. Marcus Bent adores Davina McCall but I never got it myself. Styled by blind nuns. Davina, not Marcus.

It gets worse. The cries for help from my left hamstring are overridden by howls of complaint from my lower back and also from my right groin, which has never had a mind of its own. Various areas are clearly working in cahoots to bring about a timely end to this awful debacle. By the time I get to the postbox I'll be Stephen Hawking but without the brain cells. Faster on the face of it, though. Every cloud . . . if only I'd written a book that nobody understands!

My back and groin push forward a copy of the international prevention of injury treaty signed by all my body parts on the occasion of my retirement. The small print of what was basically an amnesty enables my parts to table a motion of no confidence on a majority rule basis. This motion is immediately seconded by my right knee, which in fairness has always been consistently ideologically opposed to exercise regimes.

Things are looking ominous.

As the road levels out, though, we achieve dialogue. My body has underestimated the power of the brain. My own brain is slow to get going, it stalls like an old car on a frosty morning, but once it has started to work it doesn't give up half as easily as my other muscles. My brain is a relic of what was once an ultimate fighting machine capable of extraordinary physical prowess with a will to win that made Floyd Mayweather look like a pathetic fanny. Either that or my brain has worked out that if all the other bits and pieces atrophy through laziness and lack of use it will be on its own, working out how to keep the drool off my ample bosom.

Running in pre-season is hard, really hard. There are so many things going on that affect every facet of every other thing, such as muscles and emotions. For example, if you're running as a team then you are obviously running with other people and that breeds competition to the point where some players will urge the rest of us not to set off too fast.

Let's pace ourselves, lads!

Easy does it!

Slow down, for fuck's sake!

And so on . . .

The runners in the group never listen to those anguished pleas if it's a short run. They set off at their own pace and leave the other poor bastards to hang on.

Sometimes we'd run as a squad, maybe just around the training ground, or occasionally along the river at a steady pace. Endurance running is the most mind-numbingly, physically painful and detestable exercise I know of. I'm fairly sure it is outlawed by the Geneva Convention.

This is the run I've decided to do today because it serves as a benchmark. You know where you stand with a long run, as it were – a long run will tell me just how unfit I am.

I woke up this morning knowing that I needed to do something. My heart has been hurting a lot lately and I've put it down to a chronic lack of exercise because I don't eat particularly badly. I don't eat crisps or chocolate, haven't for years, ever since Bupa came to visit us at our training ground and performed ECGs on the players and told me to cut out crisps and chocolate. My heart has hurt ever since. So much for the appliance of science.

The morning started with a series of challenges, incremental steps designed just to get me out of the front door. I decided not to shower until I got back from my run. I put on some of the clothes that Nike still send me from time to time: T-shirts, shorts and trainers, though no socks. No problem. There is a dedicated drawer in my bedroom (and I suspect every other footballer has one) filled with kit from a number of clubs that I've played for over the years. Trust me, socks aren't a problem. At football clubs, kit goes missing like a foreign number 10 on a cold Tuesday night at Stoke.

Once a year, the kitman holds a kit amnesty that allows the players to bring back all of the kit they have taken home, without receiving a fine for taking it in the first place. The mountain that appears on the changing-room floor the following morning could clothe Africa. Believe me, all Geldof has to do is visit Premier League football clubs at certain times of the year and he'd never need to bother another ageing rock star again.

So now I'm dressed and out. First tasks ticked off the list.

Not too out of breath either. Despite the pain, I am impressed with myself – although, being honest, I am impressed with myself any day I succeed in getting out of bed before noon. Today I arose with consummate ease at 10.30 a.m. Still got it. Is this exercise nonsense really necessary? I'm a Gurkha at heart.

I came downstairs and had a black coffee. That usually gets the tubes working. For those of you who have wondered, I'm very regular, but this morning nothing happened. I was nervous and tight inside and I also cursed myself for forgetting to buy half a dozen lemons the day before, one of which would have gone into a pint of lukewarm water to be downed on the spot. A pint of warm water and the juice of a lemon is the first thing any fitness geek should have in the morning as it speeds up the metabolism and burns the fuel in your body faster. For the same reason, I didn't have anything to eat for breakfast. I was to embark on a run aimed at incinerating the fat stored by my body, not the energy from a bowl of muesli.

It occurred to me that timekeeping might be a problem. I don't own a Fitbit. Maybe I should postpone all manoeuvres until I have one. Fact is, I'm still stalling at the gate with the Fitbit move. They are pretty useful gadgets but I just don't want to be a Fitbit Wanker because that makes me like all those people who go to gyms just to show off their Fitbits. If I'm running it will be on my terms, preferably with as few people doubled over laughing at me as possible. Anyway, I'm so old and slow most measurements of speed and distance could be taken using a sundial.

Because I don't own a Fitbit, I don't know how far my route actually is, but I do know where I'm going. I'm heading out of my country road, down the main road, into and around the field earmarked for housing, and back again. I estimate that it's approximately the same as running from John O'Groats to Land's End. I'm using the field because it's softer than the road. My knees aren't built for road running. They hurt just walking up the stairs, but Mrs TSF won't let me invest in one of those chair lifts for the elderly.

Without a Fitbit I needed some kind of timekeeping device though. I was reluctant to take my phone, although it did offer the hope of somebody using GPS to locate my lifeless body if this running lark proved as dangerous as I feared. I looked around and spotted my son's watch, bought with his birthday money from Smiggle, which tells the time in giant red electronic numbers. Perfect. That brought me another step closer to the door and possible fashion immortality.

But then I got cocky. I remembered that about six years ago I stole two 10kg arm weights from the gym of a Premier League club I played for. I told myself that I'd do some arm weights when I got back, possibly even some core exercises. I found them in the garage where they'd survived every attempt by my wife to spring-clean. She's obviously been trying to tell me something. I picked the first one up and almost dislocated my shoulder. I thought Mrs TSF had been walking funny since 2010. I'd assumed the blame lay with our firstborn. She'd obviously tried lifting one of these girders.

How did I ever steal them without help? Why did I steal them? How had I thought they were 10kg weights when obviously they are easily 30kg apiece? I rolled them to an appropriately shaded place in the garden, convincing myself that I'd hit them as soon as I got back. Or they'd make for an unusual piece of conceptual landscape gardening.

Back to the mutiny of my muscles. The dull ache is still there, bitching about the whole fitness deal. I make it to the main road. Gentle undulations rather than peaks and valleys, and as my mind clears I have an idea. It's a good one, and I tell myself not to forget it whatever happens. It requires me to make a note on my phone and then a call when I get home (after the weights and the core exercises obviously). Why didn't I bring my phone? I could stop and do it now and walk for a bit while I chatted.

My heart is beginning to hurt.

Not my head. Please.

I keep going but I'm beginning to wonder if I shouldn't stop all this health stuff now – for health reasons. My heart is pounding out of my chest. My legs feel as though somebody has removed my torso and poured concrete through the tops of them. I can't move.

My heart dithers for a while, wondering whether to give up, but then it breaks into some kind of rhythm. I try to remember the pace I ran at when I was in my prime. It was much faster than this, that I do know. It must have been. Surely? I wasn't the fastest but I wasn't the slowest either. Mine was a perfectly acceptable Premier League pace and, most importantly, it maxed my heart rate: in training, we would all wear heart-rate monitors that told the sports scientist via a laptop set up at the side of the pitch, in crude terms, whether or not we were trying our hardest.

They do this by taking readings for the player's active heart rate and his resting heart rate and by measuring the time that it takes to recover after exercise. The thing to remember about any run during training is that you usually have to do three laps of the football pitch, three times over. You get a minute's rest between each set so it pays to finish each one as quickly as you can so that you get more rest. Faster runners get the full minute while the less fit players have only twenty or thirty seconds before they have to set off again.

I don't need a heart-rate monitor now to tell me that I feel like shit. Running on the road is killing my knees and the temperature is soaring. It feels like pre-season all over again – except with nothing to look forward to. I see the field up ahead and it has a push-me-pull-you gate. That gate is a little oasis. Obviously I can't run through it; I need to stop for a bit in order to pull the gate towards me and step around it. Seven steps of pure sanctuary.

As I set off again I notice that the field is overgrown with that grass that whips your shins with surprising accuracy and determination. I also notice that this is a bloody big field. The council has offered it up to the government as part of its commitment to allocate plots of brownfield land for housing, and the planning application is showing nine hundred houses, a small village square with room for a Tesco Express and a collection of luxury apartments that stand no chance of ever getting past the Trade Descriptions Act. Yes, it's a big field.

The slightest little thing that puts you off your rhythm makes the run so much harder: stepping up on to the pavement from the road, having to sidestep some dog shit, even waving away a fly, or putting your foot on an uneven part of the ground and losing your balance. Anything that means you have to adjust your breathing makes it harder to find the flow again.

In pre-season these kinds of problems didn't exist. No. The problem in pre-season was running with someone who wanted to talk to you. Talking is probably the worst thing you can do while running: it completely ruins your breathing pattern, slows you down as a result – and you may get a smack in the face from me. For your own sake, don't talk to me.

I make my way around the field (or rolling prairie). It's peaceful – the diggers won't arrive for a couple of years – and in spite of the grass lacerating my shins I have managed to find a rhythm. It mostly involves me breathing out of my arse but it's a start.

Just then a pigeon hurls itself into the air and scatters half a dozen of its mates on various trajectories away from me. It is one of nature's great mysteries, how a pigeon can make more noise than an Airbus A380 the moment it chooses to leap from its branch and fly away. Startled, I turn to look at the commotion and veer off the path. My legs immediately tighten, which upsets my back and messes with my breathing to the point that I cough up what turns out to be bile. For a moment I face the prospect of the Great One-Year Health Plan being derailed on day one by pigeons.

My brain has a trick up its sleeve though (if brains have sleeves). It daydreams. This may sound like a bad thing but it isn't, it's a glorious thing. I used to do it while I was running in pre-season.

In the Premier League the cream rises to the top, physiologically: players with better physical attributes who are also talented wind up playing there. Sounds obvious. As a consequence, the running in the Premier League pre-season is far harder than in the lower leagues. In my experience, players are simply able to cope with more and so they are fitter and stronger and get asked to cope with even more. On the pitch during games I was very fit. I chased everything and everyone and was still able to do the extra stuff that wasn't necessarily what was expected of me. That fitness was built up during pre-season, but there were far better runners and far fitter players than me. I needed to find some trick that let me compete so that I could enjoy the same level of fitness on the pitch when the season started. Daydreaming was my secret weapon. My brain was able to carry me through pain barriers just by drifting off.

I'll give you an example.

A favourite test of sports scientists, or fitness coaches, is to have you run around the pitch three times as fast as you can. Sounds easy. It absolutely isn't. You need a plan to get through those three laps and it goes like this: use adrenalin to get through the first lap, pace yourself in the second lap, and hang on for the last lap.

My system was roughly the same, except on the middle lap I just drifted off. I allowed my brain to wander and before I knew it my attention had been taken off the pain of the task. Other lads were wheezing but I was thinking about what I had to buy at Sainsbury's later on. I'd visualize the aisle, imagine the soft but shit background music, and in my mind I'd be wandering around the supermarket. Two laps gone, just like that. When your brain switches back to reality you wonder how you got the last lap done. Anyone can do it, indeed I bet many of you do. Imagine you are in your car: you drive to the shops and before you know it you've arrived. You can't remember any part of the journey or anything about changing gear or braking and steering; you can't even remember what the traffic was like. Same thing. It's called the 'subconscious mind'.

For the first time I consider the distance I have left to run. It seems vast, but it isn't, maybe a mile, but it is mostly uphill, with a final ascent to my house. My legs tighten.

In desperation I ask my brain to dredge up something about how to cope with distance running. I rummage through old memories of pain and breathlessness but it's been too long. The best I come up with is an 'Idiot's Guide to Psychology'. It tells me about:

1. The Pratfall Effect: *your likeability will increase if you aren't perfect.*
    Bullshit.
2. The Bystander Effect: *the more people that see you in need, the less likely you will receive their help.*
    We'll see when I collapse in the fucking road and get hit by a cement mixer.
3. The Spotlight Effect: *your mistakes are not noticed as much as you think.*
    I got sent off in front of a crowd of 75,000 once. Trust me, even the section for the blind and partially sighted noticed that.
4. The Paradox of Choice: *the more choices we have, the less likely that we'll be happy with our decision.*
    There are only two options here, live or die, and if I make it back to the house and live to tell the tale, believe me, I'm going to be the happiest man since Happy McHappy invented the Happy Meal in Happy Town.

5. The Focusing Effect: *people place too much importance on one aspect of an event and fail to recognize other factors.*

Yes! That's it! It all comes back to me as I finish my circuit of the field and enjoy the seven steps through the push-me-pull-you gate once more.

Running in pre-season, I had to concentrate on where other players were and listen out for the times being shouted out periodically by the fitness coach. Certain things happened that panicked me, broke my concentration, hurt me, annoyed me, and generally served to put me off my stride and make me more tired. To deal with those things my brain conjured up a series of 'blocks'.

For example, if my legs hurt, my brain calculated the distance I had left to run in an instant. Unfortunately, it could be a distance that my body couldn't cope with, so my legs felt even heavier. My brain would then try again. 'Just make it to that cone,' it said, 'then to the next pole, then round that last cone – come on, you're almost there.' The whole run was broken down into manageable chunks – like me cutting up my son's sausages.

My run now becomes a war of attrition. I just need to make it past that V W Camper Van. Then I need to get to the spooky tree on the corner without suffering a cardiac arrest. Next is the kink in the road, and finally the top of the last hill. Make that climb and I'll be Rocky. I'll shuffle home with my arms raised over my head. My own greatest hero.

Why did I buy a house on a fucking hill? The hill almost finishes me off but I'm so close to home that I know now somebody will find me if I collapse in a mangled heap. That's how close I feel to being Rocky. Just to the end of the tarmac right before the road turns to gravel and then to the crossroads that veers up towards a neighbour I haven't seen in about five years. Maybe he went for a run one day and never came back. Maybe he'll be peeping out of his window looking at me going past in apparent slow motion while he says to himself, 'Christ, poor Mr TSF got old fast.'

I make it past each landmark. Suddenly I'm staring down the barrel of the sweetest victory since an astonishing win over Arsenal that, as a Spurs fan, I still get an enormous kick out of.

As a player, you would usually make a final sprint for the line, just like a track runner at the Olympics. This isn't to improve your time necessarily, it's because this is the part of the run when your body is working hardest and it will therefore benefit the most from a last spurt of energy, whether that means putting some extra stamina in the bank or making a withdrawal of fat.

I try to give it a last push but the body has nothing left to give, which is a good sign. I keep my pace and make it to the front door, banging it with my hand in triumph. It is an extraordinary achievement, right up there with Leicester's Premier League title and Iceland's victory over England at Euro 2016. Astonishing.

There's a commentary loop screaming in my head. He's done it! He's done it! The veteran has rolled back the years! Grit, determination, bloody-mindedness! One of the greatest moments in sporting history!

I fall through the door and every fibre of my being is telling me to reach for an ice-cold can of Coke – left over from Christmas, before you ask – but I resist gallantly and pour myself a pint of lukewarm water.

Then the unsteadiness arrives. There is a slight dizziness, and I see flashing circular lights everywhere I look. They weren't there earlier. I teeter from the kitchen towards the lounge but have to break for the downstairs loo door where I just about manage to get the toilet lid up (why does she always put it down?) before I deposit one pint of lukewarm water, one cup of black coffee and half my stomach lining. That's not carrot, kids, it's actually your stomach lining, and it doesn't grow back.

I have to sit down. I'm afraid though. Afraid of stiffening up and contracting into something the size of a golf ball. If I close my eyes I may die. Or is that when you have concussion? Who knows. I may just die anyway. Mrs TSF will be so sorry she laughed at me.

I recall the time-honoured cool-down that states players must immediately fill their body with protein – which I don't – and then lie on their backs with their legs up a wall at a right angle. The idea is to drain all the lactic acid out of your legs towards the heart which will pump it around the body until it is sufficiently dispersed.

I'm only too happy to try the lying down bit. I choose the lounge floor and wall because from there I can at least see the TV. If I flick the channels maybe I'll find somebody who is actually training for, say, the London Marathon. I'll laugh at them – if it doesn't hurt too much.

As I'm lying there with my heart pounding and head throbbing and cramp spasms sprinting up and down my legs, I notice my mobile phone on the coffee table. What ensues is a full two-minute battle to reach it. It takes me those two minutes to see that on the other side of me is a kitchen roll tube my son has been using as a telescope. (Have you seen the price of the real ones? It's not like he's going to discover a new galaxy.) I grab it and use it to manoeuvre my phone towards me.

I pick it up, dial a number, and a familiar voice answers straight away.

'Hello mate,' he says, 'long time. You sound out of breath. You fallen off your bar stool again? I'm just going into training – some of the lads were injured in the Euros – but what can I do for you?'

I breathe deeply and slowly. Compose myself.

'Well, two things, mate. First of all, I had a good idea while I was running.'

'What was that? Never to run ever again?'

'No mate. Do you want to write a book together?'

'Hmmm. What was the second idea?'

'Well, can you drop in and put my body back together when you're finished with those losers? I actually think I'm dying.'

'Sounds interesting,' says The Secret Physio. 'See you this afternoon.'

And that he did.

I was still on the lounge floor when he arrived, like a weird discovery at Pompeii but minus the solidified ash. Yet.

The Secret Physio agreed to do the book. And what follows is a typical year in the life of a Premier League club from the perspective of What the Physio Saw. And it is just that – a typical season, not one particular season but a whole load of stories from throughout his time as a Premier League physio. I'll be chipping in what I've called my Second Opinions so he doesn't get too much of my limelight . . .

JULY

H ere we go again . . .
Football finishes. Then football catches its breath. Cue
hype. Then football starts all over again. The team that finished on top of the mountain the previous May is at base camp
now. So are all the also-rans. The period between those climbs
is holiday time.

For me as a physio, football holidays are both too long and
too short. Too long for players. Too short for me. Maybe I have
just been doing this for too long.

Today is the start of pre-season, a time of blood, sweat and
tears. Mainly sweat. A few of the players, mainly the old lags,
have been haunting the training ground for a week or so now,
hoping to get a head start because they know what is coming
and how their limbs will protest about it. There's one or two
who are wishing they'd looked after themselves better back in
the day and sense that the end is nigh. There's a few more who
will be getting contracts into their mid-thirties: you take good
care of the engine, you get better mileage.

This morning, the old guys sense the rushing sounds of time

passing quickly. The place is flooded with young guys with fresh tans, new haircuts and spine-chilling war stories from their holidays. There's the odd new transfer as well, quietly trying to fit in.

I look at the old crew, the stalwarts and the veterans (as the newspapers might call them), and I can read their thoughts. 'I just had a quiet holiday with the missus and the kids,' they're thinking. 'I played a little golf and I ate more salad than I ever thought was possible. And like a good pro I came back here a week ago to kick-start my pre-season. But I still feel like shit! Everything aches. Every muscle groans. I spend more time getting massages than I do actually working on the field. And now the place is full of these feckless youngsters with more money than sense. Way more money. And they've spent the summer drinking and debauching. And they are raring to go. I hate them.'

We have a new manager who will be introducing himself to us some time today. Last season we scraped into the Champions League, which sounds like success for most clubs, but it was failure for us. The old manager had been a dead man walking since the team lost four games on the trot. We dropped from being title contenders to the subject of all those 'Where has it all gone wrong?' articles that pundits love so much.

The season finished and we never saw our old manager again. He got the bullet. A nice gold bullet that paid him in full for the two years he had left on his contract. Both parties wished the other well and told the media that the relationship had been ended by mutual agreement. Not a bullet. Not at all. A conscious uncoupling.

So we have a new guy, and all the pressure in the world is on him. In football, pressure trickles downhill. We hope he handles it well.

There is no sense of certainty around the club at the moment. There never is when you go into a new season with new management. Apart from hoping that nobody will lose their jobs, the other anxiety about a new regime is that they might turn out to be cliquey and stand-offish. We've had managers and coaches here before who have been very distant, and an 'us and them' mentality has set in.

This new lot are rumoured to be very sociable though. The advance members of the new coaching staff we have met have been overly open and friendly, and it has been very easy to talk to them informally and get a picture of where we are all going.

In my experience at top clubs I have never really found myself being dictated to. New coaches have generally been keen to see how the current medical department is run. They have then left us to do our thing.

They might want more influence when a player is getting back to fitness. Our last manager was very open to modifying training. If a player was 70, 80 per cent fit but not capable yet of doing certain things in training, he was still happy for that player to train and avoid doing those things. That will change in the upcoming season. If a player can't do everything, if he isn't 100 per cent fit, he won't train with the first team. My training is my training. I don't change my training for anybody. I don't want a player breaking down. We have to make sure that we keep a player long enough so that when he goes back in he is 100 per cent immersed without danger to himself.

To be honest, we have such fantastic facilities at the top clubs it is hard to screw things up. The shit only hits the fan when you mess up a particular player, or the management of a particular player. Things can go wrong with a complicated or nasty injury. That is when managers get a bit more twitchy and unhappy. If you tell them a player will be back in four weeks, and four months later the player is still not back, they get very uncomfortable and start questioning how good their medical team is.

At the start of pre-season, the staff tend to drift towards the training ground in dribs and drabs. Sometimes, you might meet the fitness coach four or five days before everyone else to see if he needs more equipment, changes to the gym. The manager himself comes in a few days before all the players, just to say hello and, if necessary, introduce himself. Usually you have a few players in who were struggling with injuries towards the end of the previous season and have set up a second home in the training-ground gym to try to get a jump on their teammates. The older ones especially see the benefits of getting the achy bones and joints out and oiled up before the young whippersnappers come back.

At top clubs, if you had players at a summer tournament then you may only have 30 per cent of your first-team squad at the start of pre-season. To make the numbers up to twenty-five or thirty players, the coaches will pick out some youngsters to train with the main group. As the older 'international' first-teamers come back from their holidays and join the group, the young lads get released back to the youth team. It seems a little cruel but it is a good window for them to make an impression on management before the season starts.

By the way, can somebody remind me why we give players the best part of two months off at the end of a season? For most clubs the close of business comes in mid-May, and if there is no World Cup or European Championship all players are granted six to seven weeks' shore leave. Off they go, scattered to the most expensive corners of the Earth with no mandatory training or conditioning work to do.

Whatever resentments the old players might have – the Jurassic Park crew as I call them – the young players who have ambled back in here this morning aren't as fit as they might look. A couple of kilos' worth of excess baggage being carried around the midriff might not be visible to the layman, but for an elite athlete it means running slower and becoming fatigued faster. They look like a bunch of millionaire athletes all right, but when I watch them out on the training field it is all too plain to see that many of them have lost conditioning. They'll have to embark on a six-week schedule with double sessions thrown in for extra fun. That's what pre-season is all about. Penance, suffering and getting fit enough to be part of the plans that are being drawn up.

For most clubs, pre-season involves eight or nine games played at lower-level grounds against players who are desperate to show off and claim a higher-league scalp. Or maybe to leave a scar on a Premier League leg. In recent years, thanks to multinational sponsors, bigger clubs like ours have taken to flying abroad and playing other big clubs in lucrative friendly games dressed up as 'mini-tournaments'. That involves a lot of air miles for players and staff who already travel a lot anyway, and the intense work has to continue wherever the team is. Sometimes it's fine. Sometimes you fly to Beijing, as Manchester United have done, and discover that the pitch in the Bird's Nest stadium is about as suitable for football as, well, a bird's nest. So you fly straight back home again and call your lawyers and insurance carriers.

It's a recipe for six weeks of stiff muscles, constant tiredness, blisters, long days and grumpy men.

I know this is unlikely to catch on as an idea among players, but having only three weeks off would actually be better for them. Your thoroughbred athletes will not decondition that much in three weeks. And if we took three weeks off in the summer we could have a fortnight break early in the new year and spread some of the load in the fixture list.

Or . . .

Why don't teams just do something revolutionary, like give players two weeks of complete rest at the end of the season to mentally and physiologically recharge their batteries? Then come in for three or four medium-intensity sessions, then have another two weeks with three maintenance (conditioning) sessions to do. Then they'd return to the regular 'pre-season' period in a lot better shape. It would be less punishing, the injury rate would decline, and there surely couldn't be too many complaints from guys earning £200,000 a week. There would be no necessity to embark on an intensive training schedule like boot camp recruits getting ready for a long war.

A few managers have tried to do things differently but there has been no consistency. Football is very traditional. We hate change, even if it makes physiological sense.

It would make more sense for England too. I'm not sure what Gareth Southgate thinks but I know that his ill-fated predecessor Sam Allardyce was a fan of the restructured season. We'll see. Maybe Sam has just been around too many relegation-haunted teams. A winter break when you are struggling is a respite from all the pressures.

Look at it this way. I think I would win the argument if somebody went away and made a study of those top players who need to perform consistently for their club during the season and who play international tournaments most summers and who then get only two or three weeks off before returning for pre-season.

This morning, though, nobody wants to listen to the physio's enlightened theories on how the game should be run. The players hovering around the medical room are telling their stories of the summer. I listen to hair-raising anecdotes and scandalous dispatches from Dubai, Miami, Bali and beyond.

These players spend more on a holiday than most of us staff earn in a year. Personally, when summer comes around I like to find a nice quiet village somewhere in Spain or France, chill out with the family and pretend that football doesn't exist. That means I don't have many stories of my own to trade, but it's fun to listen to their exploits, especially the younger guys. The medical staff exchange quick amused glances as we give leg rubs and look for the source of new-found niggles and pains. These boys are going to suffer for those excesses over the next few weeks! Penance and purge, lads.

This morning, the right full-back's missus isn't talking to him. He holidayed with the lads in May and completely blew his end-of-season bonus (think of the current market price of your house). Then he went to France on another jolly, so, in short, he wasn't at home much. Hell hath no fury like an ignored WAG. And his hamstring has been nagging him too.

Our player, who had a bad season last year, continued his run. He fell in love with a woman and in one wonderful night they tripped the light fantastic of all the clubs and sights. She shook him awake in the morning. She needed $10,000. Or else. He paid. Later he discovered that his Rolex was missing, along with his dignity.

'You were in Vegas. Did you not suspect anything?'

'No. I thought I loved her.'

'OK. And now you want us to check you for STDs?'

'Is that OK?'

We deal with all sorts in the medical room. There are the hypochondriacs ('I just have a real bad feeling about my left knee'), the old soldiers ('Actually your knee is cratered and soft like a Swiss cheese – we're going to have to manage it carefully') and the usual suspects with their hamstrings, dodgy calves, weak ankles and treacherous backs.

Take a ticket and form an orderly queue.

The new manager has just walked into the medical room with his assistant and that woman from the office who always accompanies new managers on their first day. He's the latest in a long line of coaches brought in to achieve the impossible dream since I've been here. I know the routine by now. It's like standing in line to meet a royal but with more serious consequences if you fail to observe etiquette.

There is a slightly awkward moment before we all realize that the new manager is among us and we must stop whatever it is that we are doing. We manage this just before the woman from the office embarrasses herself and claps her hands for our attention as if we were schoolchildren.

We walk towards the new man and his assistant, who looks as though he will definitely be the mean one in any good cop/bad cop routine. We introduce ourselves one by one, giving our job titles as we do so. Not that he'll remember us all in five minutes but it seems like the thing to do.

His CV is impressive and he must have been through this routine at just about every club he has ever managed. Still, I reckon he looks a little bit more nervous than we are. There is a reason for this.

There was a time, again back in the Middle Ages when I started in football and we used to cut players' limbs off with rusty saws, when a manager's medical team was one overworked physio. The manager often thought he knew a lot more than that physio. So a new manager coming into a club often meant that the poor overworked physio was one of the limbs that got sawn off the payroll straight away. The manager might even bring his own physio with him.

At smaller lower-league clubs today there may still be only one physio and they will have a very close working relationship with the manager – if they don't, they will be out of a job. I know. I have been that physio. Back in the days when I was the sole first-team physio at a small club, whenever a new manager came in I would feel uncertain about my future. It was up to me to prove to him that I could provide an efficient medical service. I also had to hope that he recognized an efficient medical service when he saw one – and that he wasn't dragging a mate/ physio with him from club to club.

This has all changed. Today us medical geeks have fewer worries as we set about our work for pre-season. We need to make a good impression – and good communication is essential to us doing our jobs well – but we were here before the current manager, and because we do our jobs well we will be here after he's gone. For us, a change of manager is a case of 'the king is dead, long live the king'. We are the civil service. Ruling parties come and go. We go on until we retire. Or until we accidentally kill somebody.

At the larger clubs (with larger medical teams), we physios have become something of a protected species. There will be a head of department who will usually be either a doctor or a physiotherapist and who falls under the control of the board of directors. Some of the top Premier League clubs, including ours, now have four to five first-team physios; even many Championship clubs have two or three, each with their own speciality.

Contracts for the medical staff don't necessarily follow those of the manager. They are organized separately and independently. So things change, but by and large our professional lives remain the same. Our club, for instance, has spent millions on its training-ground facilities and the cost of the medical department absorbed many of those millions. In the department we have staff who have been carefully recruited from all over the world and who have a store of knowledge not just about their own speciality but about the players at the club, how they respond to various treatments, and what their weaknesses are.

We earn good wages and we generally have close ties with the players – as do most physios at any club – therefore changing medical staff can be disruptive and expensive. Ours is a big and successful club and the size of our medical staff reflects our status. The average Premier League side, say a Bournemouth or a Swansea City, will have around three physios solely dedicated to looking after the first-team squad. This, at most clubs, comprises a pool of nineteen to twenty-five players, though it can occasionally extend to thirty. The club will employ a doctor too, usually a sports medicine physician with post-graduate qualifications and experience in the field.

Where the doctor sits on the totem pole is an issue that still hasn't been fully settled. At some clubs, like Spurs (Aaron Harris) and Arsenal (Colin Lewin), a physio leads the medical department, while at others, a doctor does the job. This is the case at clubs like Manchester City (Dr Sam Erith) and Chelsea (Dr Paco Biosca). It is perceived within these clubs that the doctor holds greater status and is able to make the big decisions about players worth many millions of pounds.

Well, I have to make the case for my tribe here: this isn't always so. Most Premier League head physiotherapists have a lot more direct experience with football-related injuries, and how to manage them appropriately, than your average football team doctor.

The whole doctor/physio debate makes me feel old. Back when I started in football, the Premier League was still in its infancy and titles like 'sports medicine physician' or even 'sports doctor' had yet to be included on staff rosters. The number of doctors working at football clubs has rocketed over the past five to six years and the Premier League has facilitated this. Now, it is mandatory for all Premier League clubs to have a doctor with post-graduate sports medicine qualifications and experience available for all games.

Which is a good thing, so long as you don't find yourself working with a doctor who looks down on physios or thinks that he (or she) has nothing to learn. The day you think you know it all is the day to retire. I am a great believer in sharing knowledge and exchanging information. Doctors and physios should work together, combining differing views, approaches and opinions.

As our new manager stands among us he is faced with an intimidatingly large battalion of physiotherapists, doctors, nutritionists, masseurs, sports scientists and injury analytics experts, all stepping forward to say hello. He makes a short speech in what I already know from TV is almost perfect English.

He tells us that he has heard a lot about our good work. (Yeah, sure.)

We are very important to the club and to the team. (Who is he telling?)

We are the hidden heroes of football. (Not in our own minds.)

He'd like us to know that he appreciates everything we do. (Naturally.)

He is looking forward to working closely with us in the time to come, and he hopes that those times will be glorious. (The last three guys all said that too.)

There will be some changes for us to get used to (i.e. we will do exactly what he wants us to do or we will lose our jobs).

He has his own ways of training and preparing teams. (Oh, that's all? We won't have to be dealing with gunshot wounds or shrapnel?)

And then our new manager and his two-person entourage let us get back to work as they walk around the medical room gazing and nodding at our array of high-tech machines and gizmos.

Later in the week he will sit down with me and the lead doctor and have a general discussion about what he wants from us.

Then we'll really know what he is all about and what he expects.

Players. Players. Players. They are the ghosts in our machine. The spanners in our works. The rogue elements undermining our best-laid plans.

I was being driven by a player once to a local gym to do a session when he got so bored of going around a series of roundabouts that he drove straight over them, destroying plants and leaving tyre tracks in the grass.

Another player thought it would be amusing to put an acupuncture needle into the end of his knob and then run around the medical room showing everyone his little rifle-with-bayonet.

I've seen a player hiding in the medical room under a pile of towels while the manager came in asking if anybody had seen him. I saw the same player walk out to train in the rain minutes later wearing just his boots and socks and bollock-naked otherwise. Just for banter!

We keep a straight face through it all. Nothing surprises us about players, but unfortunately the club seems to need them. For us, dealing with players can be like trying to mind mice at a crossroads.

As they get older, thankfully they acquire some sense. Hence the greybeards coming into the training ground a week early for extra preparation.

Actually, over the years most players have got more sensible. They are being well paid during their holidays. The summer is no longer a race to see who can put the most weight on. In the old days, some clubs would announce fines for players who came back to pre-season having added a significant percentage to their body fat. Those players would come in and smack the cash down on the table before they were even tested. One club encouraged players to do some high-intensity work over the summer and gave them heart monitors, the data from which would be revealed when they came back to work. One player strapped the monitor to his dog every day while he made the mutt play fetch. The medical department weren't fooled – you K9 lovers out there will know that a dog's heart beats much faster than a human's – but they did give him injections for distemper.

Among others we've had the club captain around for the last week or so, and in fairness he is an example to the other players. Funny guy but really driven. If they all looked after themselves the way he has, especially in the second half of their careers, then they could play Premier League football almost to their mid-thirties. I don't know how many have the willpower to do that though, or the foresight to see the unavoidable damage their bodies will be suffering from years later.

The problem when it comes to the off-season is that even players with good intentions of keeping fit over the summer will pick up injuries. Then there are players who didn't have any good intentions in the first place.

Even at this level of football we have players who get by on talent alone and aren't too interested in living like elite athletes. They are good, very good, but they could be at least 10 per cent better and could play more games if they really looked after themselves.

This is football though. You can go to a country and not bother to learn the language, you can struggle with your weight and generally lose that struggle, you can fail to integrate with your team, you can have a lousy disciplinary record, but if you have a good agent and a knack for scoring goals when your backside is hovering over the bacon slicer then your next move will always be more lucrative than the last one. I'm thinking of guys like Diego Costa of Chelsea, Rayo Vallecano, Atlético Madrid (twice), Real Valladolid, Albacete, Celta de Vigo, Braga (twice) and Penafiel (as I write this). He is legendary for being his own man and being set in his ways. But there are many more. They don't adapt because they don't have to adapt. If you are good enough at football then the world will adapt around you by itself, just to keep you happy.

These are the guys who will be coming in after their holidays with all sorts of ailments that absolutely must be sorted before the season starts. When footballers are let off the reservation they are prone to almost anything. When physios talk to each other, we don't generally swap stories about hamstrings or cruciates. It's the guy who strains his hip flexor from shagging too enthusiastically, the keeper who has a large burn on his back from playing poker (his losses had mounted so he agreed to forfeits if he lost more hands, one of which involved holding a hot pan on his back for three seconds), the player who has overdosed on Viagra ('Make it go down, please'), or severed tendons in his foot after dropping something heavy on it (ironically, goalies seem most prone to this). There was one guy who had a stomach bug and somehow managed to transfer the bug to his knee. A top player once missed months of his career because he visited a friend in hospital, caught a superbug through an area of athlete's foot between his toes, and the bug burrowed into a bone in his foot.

Presenting for pre-season you have some of the damaged heroes of epic drinking, eating, gambling and rampant shagging in far-off places, and many other guys with more innocent common-or-garden ailments. I have had players coming back to the medical room in July and they've torn a cartilage playing tennis with a mate, or they've picked up a shoulder injury while they were out kayaking with the kids. Some guys have played golf every day, thus using a completely different muscle group to the ones they need for football. They come in wondering why they have back pain.

The list is endless, and the best and most interesting injuries always occur during the off-season. People are often surprised that stats show that injury rates among players are at their lowest in the final third of the season. But there is a good reason for that. By that point in the season the players are battle-hardened and their bodies are fully accustomed to the specific movements needed on the field.

So, as you can see, the rush to be fit for the new season is a stressful time. We tell them the same thing every year. Just three or four sessions in the week before 'real' pre-season commences will significantly reduce a player's stiffness – or DOMS (delayed onset muscle soreness) – and the chance of blisters.

At this time of the year, blisters can undo us. They occur when the skin experiences a sudden change. This commonly happens when players have been walking around in flip-flops for weeks on soft beaches then squeeze their feet into boots and run on grass-covered hard ground. Change of footwear and surfaces are the biggest causes, especially in pre-season when the player may have changed his boot deal or boot company and is being made to wear his sponsor's latest new design combined with playing on a variety of different pitches (hard, soft, wet, dry). Even the humid conditions in countries on tour make things worse as the foot is damper.

The best treatment for blisters is prevention. Soaking feet in surgical spirit or potassium crystals helps to dry the skin and toughen it. We also use 2nd Skin (a jelly-like covering) or Compeed (a gel plaster) over the vulnerable areas to avoid friction.

The worst case I ever saw was a player who thought it was a good idea to play basketball barefoot while he was on holiday and turned up for pre-season with four huge blisters down to raw skin. Took him a week to get his boots on again.

There is a lot of pressure on us to keep players on the field in pre-season, as that tends to be an indicator of the player's season to come. A player who gets injured in July and misses a significant part of the pre-season period has to play catch-up all season. So that first week is an essential conditioning period, especially when you have had one and a half months off.

When we sit down to talk to our new boss later this week, this will be high on the agenda.

Meanwhile, let's fix them up and get them out there.

The old lags first. When we lift the hood we know what we are looking for, where the old war wounds are, the vulnerable points, the rate of wear and tear, what sort of mileage they can expect to get from their bodies this season. They know us, and most importantly they trust us. I talk to the guys and they are comfortable telling me that the hamstring is nagging, the groin needs a rest, etc.

The new boys will have had a medical, but that procedure is not really sport-oriented. When a new player arrives we don't know his physical capacity. We don't know if he is feckless about injuries or if he is a hypochondriac who imagines every stiffness and twinge to be a sure sign of something terminal. For these first few days we are trying to find out what they are capable of and also what they are about as people.

Then there are the prodigal sons. If a player has only recently come back from an international championship, which will be the case with many of our players, they might have finished the tournament with an injury. Understandably they will have felt that they wanted to go on holiday for a couple of weeks so they won't have mentioned the injury. And then they turn up and say, 'Oh, by the way, I have a hamstring injury.'

This is problematic. If a player doesn't get the full pre-season training then invariably he will struggle throughout the campaign. It is, as I said, the crucial fitness-conditioning period. If a player doesn't complete it and reach the required level then his season will just never be the same. He won't play very much or very well, or performances will dip, or he'll have to put up with lots of niggling injuries. Every year, at all clubs, the Premier League season is littered with players who should be performing to a much higher standard but are falling below the level expected of them. Take a look to see if a player at your club was injured in pre-season. Very often you'll find the reason for below-par performances in January buried somewhere between June and July.

If the prodigals don't get past the group stage of a tournament then they will be back at their clubs at the same time as the players who stayed behind. But if they get to the knockout stages or beyond, their holiday will be delayed. Clubs try to give everybody an equal few weeks away from the game with their families. If some players have featured in the final of a championship then they may even turn up when you are on tour.

In addition, most big clubs these days have a contingent of players who are permanently out on loan. At clubs such as Manchester City and Chelsea that could well amount to more than a couple of dozen players, but most clubs (with the exception of Spurs – Pochettino is not a fan of the idea) carry a tail-end group of loanees. These range in profile from players similar in stature to Jack Wilshere and Joe Hart to younger professionals. It's a large number of people to be monitoring.

The loan players don't necessarily have to be screened but

they tend to be anyway as it gives us a chance to touch base with them. And deep down we know that nobody really takes that much care of a hire car, do they? When our players go to a club on loan, that club needs to know the player's history and any potential for problems. If they are paying his wages, or half his wages or whatever they have agreed, they don't want to sign a player who is crocked. And from our end, again it is like a hire car: we need to know what condition we are sending the player out in and what condition he is likely to come back in.

If a player has a history with a particular injury, then the club needs to know what the story is. They do their homework and ask the right questions. Sometimes when a player is signed on loan the club will conduct its own little medical. But this is usually nothing more than a box-ticking exercise that covers the physio's arse should there ever be an insurance claim down the line.

So over the first few weeks of pre-season we see them all – the old and the young, the hopeful and the doomed, the vets and the kids. Every nick and scratch gets recorded.

Whenever there is change at the top, the most interesting part for me isn't so much knowing who the new manager will be but finding out exactly when he will be showing up for work. They either come in very early and are meticulous in their planning or they leave it incredibly late. The guys who arrive late usually do so for reasons that are not their fault, for every second year there is a World Cup or a European Championship. The top guys will have been involved, either as managers or with the media.

Good luck to them, but meanwhile we are left at the training ground a week before the team is due to turn up for pre-season wondering what the plan is. Often we don't know what days we will be training or how often we will be training. The biggest challenge is getting hold of one of their fitness coaches to find out what the new man likes. You don't know if they will want to change the structure or continue what was happening before. Generally it's a mixture of the two. Our new guy has turned up late but not too late, thankfully. His entourage has been able to give us some clues.

We sat down with him this morning. There was coffee, tea and doughnuts and lots of little jokes.

Our first impressions had been good, and they were confirmed this morning. Some managers hardly talk to you; they just want the injury list and the names of those who are available and then leave you to get on with it. However, this is rare, especially when their star striker gets injured and they are yet again under pressure. They don't leave you alone!

Being left alone is probably the ideal scenario; on the other hand it's nice to have a little bit of interest and recognition from the manager. This guy seems to strike the right balance. Interested but not intrusive.

We are used to having to adapt to different management styles. Within days of meeting a new manager it is essential that we get the chance to lay out what he expects from the team physio and what he expects from the medical department. A good manager will be willing to listen to your experiences at the club and happy to see how the department runs for a while before making big changes.

That's how it went today.

If you are doing a good job and he sees that, he is unlikely to change things. In fact, he'll know that you can be of great help to him, providing feedback on players and routine practices. The physio room can be the hub of team gossip so having the physio's ear is a huge asset for a new manager. I'm not saying that we have a red phone in the medical room linking us directly to the manager's office, it's just that conversations that happen there are a good weathervane for the mood of the club or of a particular player. And it's in everybody's interest for that mood to be happy.

This afternoon we are happy.

It's July, but it's raining cats and dogs. We all know that the weather varies in different parts of the country but sometimes I think that variation is measured solely in inches of rain. Many players who have moved around the country to different clubs have commented on how it's grey and damp in the north and significantly more sunny and dry in the south. I don't know what that implies for the Midlands.

We're all familiar with the effects of too much sun but there is an increasing amount of recent evidence that a lack of sunshine can also affect your health, and an athlete's performance. I read once that Sir Alex Ferguson even went to the trouble of installing sunbeds for players at Manchester United. The plan was to give them time off during the winter months to 'soak up some rays'. They must have been a disciplined lot. I know players these days who get three days off and they fly to Dubai on a private jet. I don't think a club sunbed would be enough to convince them to stay at home.

Anyway, here's the science bit: the most efficient way of getting Vitamin D, which is an essential ingredient in cellular reactions in the immune system, bone metabolism and muscle performance, is through sunlight. A deficiency of vitamin D leads to reduced bone density (osteopenia), vulnerability to stress fractures and, in severe cases, rickets.

This is a seasonal problem. In the summer months, players have their holidays in June, they then train in July in the preseason sun (theoretically), and the season begins in the fine weather (again theoretically) of August and September, so they get their allocation via sunlight. But in the winter months, when the days are shorter and the sun weaker and not seen as often, there is a risk of insufficient exposure. A regular blood test – at our club it's every eight to twelve weeks, depending on how high-risk the player is – will identify those who have a low level of vitamin D3 in their system and we can supplement them accordingly.

So, today's grey clouds are a pre-season reminder of what is to come. Clubs can follow the Manchester United route of turning their players orange through artificial tanning beds and giving them time off to go on holiday, which the players would love. Or you can simply get outside on good-weather days and get ten to fifteen minutes of unprotected sun.

Having said that, if you live in the north-west this isn't easy.

But nothing about living in the north-west is easy, is it?

TSF: Second Opinion

The mark of a great physio

As a player I never worked with The Secret Physio. Nevertheless he is still very highly respected.

The best clubs I played for always had a great physio.

Now. Does a great physio have magical healing hands? No. Does a great physio understand your body better than you yourself understand it? No. Does a great physio give out painkillers like Smarties? No.

A great physio is a physio who will do your rehab with you. Be empathetic. He'll huff and puff along right beside you and he'll take the loneliness out of the process. There is nothing worse (well, maybe terminal illness or nuclear war) than being taken to a gym by a physio only to be told that he will be back in an hour but in the meantime you should run for fifteen minutes, row for fifteen minutes, and then have a go on the step-up machine for another fifteen minutes. All on your tod.

Physio rehab is a dish best consumed with company. When you are crocked and miserable you will be pleasantly surprised at how good you feel after beating the forty-year-old physio at every turn. Your primitive footballer brain kicks in. Mentally you are high-fiving yourself. Three times out of three you have beaten somebody who isn't a professional sportsperson and who is fifteen years older than you. The king is back!

The injury takes a back seat as you drive your body around a little bit faster than the poor old physio can drag his old bones. The best therapy/fun is the running machine. The physio will set the running machine at a pace of 17, which is tough. Your inbuilt competitiveness makes sure that you nudge the speed up gradually over the course of fifteen minutes in order to ensure that the poor bastard runs further. It's the same with the rowing machine. Make him row across the Atlantic if you can. His suffering is your recovery after all.

The beauty is that you always think you are the first, the fastest and the smartest. It couldn't possibly be the case that the physio knows exactly what is happening and is using his own suffering as a carrot to keep you moving on.

I've been at clubs where every injury is treated with a sigh and a heavy hint that all this rehab you say you have to do is very inconvenient for everybody. And you will be doing it alone. The physio won't do it with you because as we all know his paperwork won't sort itself. Apparently paperwork was his vocation back when he was young and idealistic.

Once I had what players call 'a phantom injury'. With a phantom injury your suffering is much worse because nobody believes that you are injured at all. Every physio and every scan that investigates your pain turns up the square root of fuck all as the source. Which just makes you hope that you will die in screaming pain and show them up as a bunch of cold-hearted charlatans.

The other players start to suspect that you are malingering. They make spiky little jokes with a punchline that says there is nothing wrong with you and everybody fucking knows it.

With my phantom injury I eventually went to a specialist with our physio. I'm sure our man had some sort of photoshopped qualification on the wall – City and Gilds (*sic*), that sort of thing – but he was so badly trained and so poorly versed in the Latin names for muscles and ligaments that we sat there for half an hour trying to determine what the fucking problem was. Our physio literally hadn't got the words with which to tell the specialist what was wrong with me. In the end I had to intervene helpfully and say that 'this bit here' was hurting. I'd had a previous injury to 'that bit up there'. Maybe they might be connected? The specialist was so appalled that I thought he might call social services to prevent other players suffering at the hands (or dangly bits at the end of the arms) of our physio.

In quality terms, the demography of good physios is a bit like the old Watford Gap. You get to a certain point and then, well, it all gets very grim very quickly. Watford in this case is that region that begins at around the lower half of the Championship. Physios at many clubs at that level and below have realized that they can earn more by going full-time into football than they can from slogging away in private practice. Beyond that they aren't much motivated. They recognize that the club could be doing better in terms of staffing its medical department and tracking its work but the club could be doing better at just about everything else too. They get demoralized, and even if you can cajole them into it, beating a bitter, demoralized old physio on the Nautilus rowing machine isn't that much fun after you've done it for five or six days straight.

Up yours

When I played non-league football there was a local physio who was accused of fiddling with his players. That is to say, whatever the injury to the player, its treatment always involved the physio testing the player's prostate. A finger in the rectum was apparently the precursor to diagnosing any and all ailments from a hernia to a broken femur to a gunshot wound.

He was eventually arrested and sent to prison for eighteen months. It never occurred to me to call the police when the rumours started. I was only eighteen.

I once wrote a comedy script about a hapless Sunday football team and for my physio I took 'inspiration' from this guy. It sounds sick, but consider Mr Kennedy, the teacher in *The Inbetweeners*. Same thing but bigger audience and endless repeats.

That's what concerns me the most.

Vital equipment

From the non-league Portakabin to the palatial Premier League medical centre, one piece of equipment is treasured by all. The ultrasound machine. Nobody really knows what it does but it is revered anyway. Like Her Majesty the Queen in many ways.

Physio 101. When in doubt, use the ultrasound machine. If it does nothing else, at least it works as a placebo. And when you are dealing with patients many of whom think that Placebo is a lower-league Portuguese side, that's more than enough.

The idea is that the machine emits soundwaves into the torn muscle via a smooth, round, metal instrument that is rubbed in a figure-of-eight motion over the surface of the skin. Not two zeroes or a seven. A figure of eight. The idea is that the voodoo associated with the number eight will 'encourage' the muscle fibres to bond together, thus repairing the injury. To continue the royal theme, it's like Prince Charles using some kind words to encourage his begonias to grow.

Typically this little ritual goes on for about fifteen minutes and is a waste of everybody's time. Sometimes I think I have actually heard my muscle fibres telling the ultrasound machine to just fuck off.

On one occasion our physio ran out of the gel that acts as a buffer between the skin and the cold metal instrument which administers the encouraging soundwave pulses. Using all of the wisdom he had accumulated as a lower-league physio he came up with a handy alternative. He applied Deep Heat as a gel substitute.

If this worked he was into Nobel Prize territory. By using a menthol-based pain-relieving embrocation in conjunction with a traditional ultrasound machine perhaps he could get the best out of both ends of the broom. Modestly he would tell future generations that he had revolutionized the science of healing through a mix of chance and intuition.

Sadly, the only legacy was some painful third-degree burns to our midfielder's upper thigh.

We never spoke about it ever again.

Pea hearts

A note on a little-known medical condition for which there is no cure.

There are players in football squads whom we call 'pea hearts'. That is because we are very sensitive people, and those players have small, tiny, shrivelled little hearts. They cannot be relied upon in battle. They cannot be relied upon to hold you a place in a queue at McDonald's.

'Pea heart' is a hurtful, politically incorrect label that is impossible to shake off. Once somebody calls you a pea heart you know where you stand in football. For ever. Mel Gibson made a film called *Braveheart*. Not *Bravepea*. Richard I was Richard the Lionheart. Le Coeur de Lion. Not Peaheart. Not Le Coeur de Petits Pois.

Sometimes, to the paying punters a pea heart can pass himself off as something better and more valiant. He can learn all the postures of the battle-hardened. He can throw some shapes that suggest he's right up for it. Really he's not.

The pea heart is easily spotted. The next time you are watching your favourites you can amaze and amuse your friends by keeping tabs on how some players tackle opposition players. Soon you will be able to denounce somebody as a pea heart.

Check to see if the player who obviously takes too much time with his hair only shows up for the tackles that are 70/30 in his favour. Somehow he dodges those tackles that are 70/30 the other way. He's going for it, he's going for it, but no, he's swerved away at the last second as if he just remembered he'd left an oven on somewhere near the far post.

Take a look to see if he ever gets mysteriously injured in training before a big match and tragically can't play. He's always 'gutted' because these are the matches etc., etc. Watch the theatre of his big celebration when your lot score an unlikely goal to win a game you never looked like winning. He had nothing to do with the goal but he's central to the celebration.

He's hoping that you'll remember him in that light and begin to wonder if he didn't get an assist.

He's always the last man off the pitch, dragging his war-torn body from the battlefield while somehow finding the strength to applaud the fans. He stays down longer than other players when he gets an innocuous little knock. When he finally gets up he shakes his head at the physio as if to say, 'I know I should be stretchered off but I'd rather die.' Then he hobbles for about thirty seconds, milking the moment, before trotting off to his usual hiding places. On the many days when he is injured (or carrying the burden of injury) he does local radio commentary because he is a man of the people.

'Pea heart' is, I think, the medical term, but in the dressing room the word 'shithouse' is interchangeable with it.

The official media position on the condition of peaheartedness is that it is an affliction only foreign players suffer from. The quickest diagnosis is exposure to Stoke on a cold Tuesday night.

Sad to say I have seen lots of English pea hearts. And Scottish. And Irish. Don't even get me started on the Welsh. How do they even screw up the courage to cross the Severn Bridge without having their hands held?

The truth? You can't handle the truth!

AUGUST

G ood news for the new manager! We are not planning to
assassinate him. We all agree that he has passed the medical room fitness test. He doesn't think that he knows more
than we do. It's always good when a manager knows just enough
to know that he doesn't know everything. We also saw a more
relaxed version of him on our pre-season tour, which has made
him more approachable.

A lot of people in the trade have stories of managers who feel
that what knowledge they picked up when they suffered a hamstring injury in 1982 qualifies them to critique everything that
happens in a medical room decades later. My favourite story is
the manager who insisted his centre-half, who was suffering
with a head injury, should return to action immediately and
would be fine and dandy if he was wearing a more padded
version of the Petr Cech skull cap. Two problems. He wasn't
ready to play: he was still concussed, and suffering from headaches. Secondly, he couldn't head the ball with all that soft
padding over his forehead. That fact was confirmed when the
manager lobbed up a few balls for the player. On impact with

the sponge padding, the balls produced a puffing sound like a lightly hit punchbag and then just fell rather pathetically to the floor.

There is a breed of manager, too, whose solution for everything is 'The Scan'. I've had the following conversation so many times:

Manager: He needs a scan.

Me: Well, no, I don't think—

Manager: Yeah, he needs a scan . . . we should just scan it.

Me: OK. Whatever . . .

The voice in my head is screaming, 'How the hell would you know if he needs a scan or not?' It won't change anything.

If the same player has fallen out with the manager there will be a very different conversation. Any time the player gets injured now, the manager will tell you, 'Don't mind him. It's all in his head. He's malingering.'

Me: Maybe I'll give him a scan?

Manager: What? Fuck him, don't waste your time and our money.

With managers, a little learning is a dangerous thing. I tend to go into a meeting with a new manager with an open mind and I usually expect some change to happen to my working life. I don't expect him to give me tutorials on physiotherapy.

Ideally, the medical staff at a club want a manager with an understanding of how the human body works. He should notice when players have a chronic or niggling injury. Close discussion with us where 'at-risk players' are concerned will lead to adequate rest or treatment when necessary to ensure maximum player availability. I have had to do this many times in order to keep influential senior players who are injury-prone available for games.

I have worked with over a dozen managers so I know they are all different and have their own ideas. Some like to know about every twinge, ache or pain besetting their players, whereas others only want to know when a player is not able to play. Communication can be an issue when English is not their first language but most learn quickly. After all, broken English is a dialect – at least that's what I tell myself. I fully appreciate that it is up to me to adapt to the methods of the players, not the other way round. I am here to provide a service to them, in line with the manager's style, and that's what I try to achieve.

So, there have been the know-alls who second-guess everything.

There have been the paranoids who reckon every injury is part of a plot against them. (A little learning may well be a dangerous thing but ignorance mixed with paranoia is like a ticking bomb.)

And there have been those who just left us to get on with the job. 'Perfect gentlemen' is the scientific term for this last group.

Some of this 'physiotherapy' knowledge that managers claim to possess is picked up when they complete the UEFA Pro Licence. I'm more than a bit cynical about this. A few managers have asked me to fill in the notes on their behalf for the physio part of their course. So there's a percentage of them out there who haven't actually learned anything. In fact, it's almost all of them.

Of course once a manager pays the medical room the courtesy of acknowledging that we have some form of expertise, we start looking for chances to influence that manager. To be blunt, most of the coaches' methods are based on their own experiences rather than hardcore evidence. There are stereotypical methods of doing things, such as the Italian way of lots of conditioning (running and gym work) together with football-based work. Other managers base their entire training on football. Managers become set in their ways and are convinced that what worked five years ago with one group should still work now with another group. I believe TSF once coined the term 'football moves on, one funeral at a time'.

In the medical room we know about medicine and conditioning. So just ask us!

Mind you, this is how one Premier League manager once referred to me in his half-time team talk, when the players weren't following his instructions: 'Even the fucking physio can see what is wrong and he knows fuck all about football!'

Fair enough.

The pre-season grind is fast coming to an end. I watch our lads train and wonder where we are in relation to our rivals. I've seen campaigns where not enough has been done in pre-season, a few early defeats have shaken players' confidence, and the team has spent half of the regular season trying to catch up while the fixtures rain down on them.

By now, some Premier League squads will have had ten weeks away from competitive football. One of the promoted teams will have had a couple of weeks less than that due to the play-off final. Teams with long lay-offs, such as mid-table Championship sides, will have brought their players in for a week or so at some point over the summer in an effort to minimize their deconditioning.

Much to the displeasure of the players, no doubt, but it's not like they're being waterboarded.

The players who have had the shortest off-season this year are those at clubs like ours, because they've been involved in Euro 2016. Most of the big clubs have had a player involved in the Rio Olympics as well. Generally not high-profile players (with the exception of Spurs), but all guys who will be coming back very late and will be enduring conditioning work when the season has already started. I notice that West Ham's Olympian Manuel Lanzini didn't play for Argentina in Brazil but came back to London instead for treatment for a knee injury. That's one of those 'Do you want the good news or the bad news first?' situations.

Generally the top teams in the Premier League will have had a hard time keeping tabs on their players this summer – how they are doing, and when exactly they will return. This makes preparing the pre-season period extremely difficult as not only are players turning up at different times, they're arriving in all sorts of shapes and sizes.

England's time in France was short and generally unhappy which, if I put on my club bobble hat instead of my more patriotic England retro bucket hat, is a good thing. Many of the England boys got an extra week or two off before returning to their clubs but they were all back in time to play a couple of friendlies before the season kicked off. It's not that I begrudge them time off. It's just that a good pre-season sets a player up for a good season. Every time we have had a smooth pre-season, the club has been successful. And when we have a good season we are all happier bunnies.

The Portuguese and French players who contested the Euro

final have had less time off and their condition will likely be poorer than their fellow players', simply from coming off the back of a long Premier League season and then a tournament. Even if they got no game time in France they will have needed a rest and a holiday after the championship.

If any of our players carried an injury through the tournament, we're unlikely to have heard about it from the player or his national team. Players don't want to be brought in early for treatment or rehabilitation. And their national team's medical staff have their own pressures to cope with to get the players to play and perform. They have no long-term or even mid-term concerns. When a player is with his national team at a major international tournament, that national team's priority is simply to get him through the duration of that tournament. Which is why we get players back who sheepishly admit that they are going to need treatment before they can train fully.

I'll be keeping an eye on the French players in particular when the season starts. Ten of France's squad were from the Premier League. How much can we expect from guys like Yohan Cabaye, Dimitri Payet, Anthony Martial, Morgan Schneiderlin, Moussa Sissoko, Bacary Sagna, N'Golo Kanté and others? Surprisingly (or not, depending on how you view the Premier League), the Portuguese only took two Premier League players with them and they both played for Southampton (José Fonte and Cédric Soares).

Liverpool had twelve of their squad at the Euros, Spurs and United eleven players each, Arsenal sent eight, and every club that competed in the league last season sent at least one player. I worry for Liverpool in particular, and will be interested to watch how Jürgen Klopp handles the season. In Germany he had some success but there was criticism that his teams faded as the campaign went on and their high-intensity pressing game wore them down. With a disrupted pre-season and no winter break in England, will he change the game plan a little for 2016-17?

I do wonder sometimes if the objective of preparing players properly for the season has become a secondary one. Take the tours we went on. During the pre-season the team took off for a trip around Denmark and Sweden. I didn't go, thankfully. I'm not really at home very much once the season gets into full swing so I'd rather not have to spend too much of the summer on the road as well.

Big clubs always go abroad in the summer these days. The Premier League is such a colossal worldwide brand that it pays clubs to go out there and milk it. Liverpool have gone after the Australian market big time so they tend to go down under quite regularly. Chelsea like to go to America and Asia on alternate years. City and Tottenham have their own markets. Even Southampton have big links in the Baltimore/Washington area. The Premier League is a massive global juggernaut. Clubs you wouldn't expect to be going far afield are now heading out, grabbing a slice of the action. Our lot came back from this European jaunt, then a few days later everybody was off abroad again for a couple of weeks. By the time we got back, the season's opening fixture was less than a fortnight away.

West Ham's pre-season schedule was even more punishing. I didn't envy them. Starting from 6 July, they had two games in the States, then three games in Austria, then a Europa League qualifying game in Slovenia before playing two games in three days at home: the second leg of their Europa League tie and a friendly against Juventus. That's a lot of time on the road for a pre-season, and again I'm wondering how it will affect a club trying to settle into a new stadium.

Playing a lot of football is a good thing for players' conditioning, but at this time of year you do need to lay the foundations with some fitness work. This can be done on the road, but a lot of travel puts pressure on players. Variations in climate, poor training surfaces, inadequate training facilities, and unfamiliar hotels and beds are all changes that an already tired, deconditioned player must deal with.

You would think that when these tours are organized the clubs would ensure that their players are going to be in the best environment with the best facilities, with a great match schedule against stimulating opposition, in order that they can then fly home and embark on a successful league campaign. But no. The theory and the practice are very different. It's usually the marketing department of the club that takes the lead when it comes to touring, and their decisions are based on where they feel the club will sell the most merchandise in order to increase profits.

As a result, you are often playing and training on surfaces that are terrible. We've played on pitches that have been converted from a baseball field into a soccer pitch, but with the mound still left in the middle. Temperatures can be horrendous. You spend much of your time dealing with dehydrated players. We have been on Asian tours where the heat and humidity have been unbearable. It can't be healthy. I wouldn't mind if we were based in Dubai for a season, then it might make some sense. But how is this good prep for Manchester on a cold Saturday afternoon, or Stoke on those famous Arctic Tuesday nights?

When Manchester United flew into Beijing that time, a bit of advance research might have told the club that the pitch at the Bird's Nest stadium was unplayable. Instead, it was a commercial disaster that cost not only a fortune but a few valuable days of pre-season. Everything was packed up and flown there and the players ended up sitting on the planes stewing in uncertainty for far longer than was necessary. I've never seen a big correlation between miles travelled and a team's performance early in the season but I suspect that missing three days of pre-season like that took a little bit out of United. And it makes everybody look bad. Players put themselves into their clubs' hands as trustingly as babies. If they are flown to Beijing and then flown back again because the pitch is unplayable they will get the sense that somebody, somewhere, has messed up.

What's the best thing for the team doesn't always come first. The medical department doesn't get involved but I would love to be in on the discussions about what is right for the team and what is right for the club commercially. Obviously growing the brand and selling the merchandise is beneficial for the club, but the club being successful and winning trophies increases its profile. Who has a larger fan base, Manchester United or Everton? Who has been more successful in terms of silverware?

Football is becoming increasingly popular in Asia so that's where the bigger clubs tend to go nowadays (although newly promoted Middlesbrough went on a good old-fashioned jaunt to Marbella, I noticed). It's a logistical nightmare, though, as we have to take the proverbial kitchen sink with us in order to provide as good a medical service as we would back home and cover every possible eventuality in even the remotest locations. Many club physios have a similar experience to the players when they go on tour for ten to fourteen days during pre-season. No days off, no family, living in hotels, in an unfamiliar climate and culture, with organized games every three days.

Do you feel our pain?

In addition to the heat and humidity, extra challenges for the staff and players include mosquitoes, an unfamiliar diet – despite the club chef bringing the ketchup, Marmite and other home comforts – and fanatical fans. Even adapting to travel itself is a skill that top players have to learn. Generally, players are used to sleeping in different beds and travelling to hotels and having that rhythm to their lives. But you usually take a very mixed squad, including a few of the youth team as some of the first-team squad may still be on holiday or injured, or simply because the coach wants to take a look at them. Players with only lower-league experience might sleep in their own beds overnight regularly, and wouldn't have gone to a hotel the night before matches because their club couldn't afford that expense, unlike most Premier League teams. If these players suddenly go on one of these tours they might have problems for a while. International players are the most gifted at coping – they can sleep anywhere.

Injured players don't tend to travel, so while the reserve/first-team squad was in Europe I stayed behind to look after them. For me that was also, as I said, a chance to work normal hours while the kids were still on holidays. The season itself is so busy that being away in the summer period isn't something us family guys look forward to. I did go on the second tour, though, because there were more first-team players on that one.

Some days during pre-season we start at eight in the morning and don't finish until eight at night. It can go on even later when you're on tour as players know you're free and they get a bit bored. Most days include double training sessions. They might train at ten in the morning and again at three in the afternoon, having gone off to do some commercial gig in between times, or just to chill at home or in a nearby hotel. You are getting them ready from early on and bringing them down for a few hours after they finish, tending to this ache and that niggle all the while. By early August you're on your knees praying for the start of the season.

On tour, the team might play a game every three or four days against a few big clubs whose pre-season paths or commercial interests have been designed to intersect with your own. There are lots of meetings and other responsibilities for the players to commit to. We also play lower-league teams as it can generate some valuable income for them. The facilities are usually less glamorous than what we have come to expect at the top level but I love it as it reminds me of my early days in the job. It makes me laugh watching a squad of twenty-four Premier League players have to change in rotation as there isn't enough space in the dressing room. Not to mention watching the kitman get stressed because he has no room for the twenty skips of kit he has to bring.

Players are always heading off during the day right through the tour period no matter where you are or what country you are in. Photo opportunities, press conferences, fan days, the harvesting of freebies that they don't really want but grab greedily anyway. Players are a stingy bunch mostly and love a freebie.

You could be in one city for two days and then move somewhere else. Sometimes in Asia or America you might get the chance to be based close to a large college facility in or near a major city and the set-up will be decent. Not having to ship out and pack everything away every couple of days is a bonus. It is nice to get a bit of routine instead of coming home from a trip and only being able to recall lugging gear all over the place for a couple of weeks.

And as I said earlier, we really do have to take that medical kitchen sink. We travel prepared for anything from a heart attack and a broken neck to a concussion, broken legs and pelvic fractures. We take *everything*. You have to have enough to cover every training session – and there might be sixteen of them – and five games. And that's half a dozen skips' worth of gear. Crutches, tape, saline, lotions, splints and defibrillators, ready for any emergency. We also take electrical machines for treatment such as ice compression machines, muscle stimulators and ultrasound devices, to help speed up the healing process. The only thing we don't take is oxygen and Entonox (nitrous oxide) because you can't take these on the plane. When you arrive you must source these things locally.

For a few players who have problems with neck or back we even bring pillows. We've had players who ended up sleeping on the floor because they couldn't cope with the beds. Sometimes a player's bed at home can't be replicated anywhere else, so the floor is the closest thing for him.

We have to organize an ambulance and paramedics to be available for every training session in case there is an emergency. You have to find out where the nearest hospital is and what the quickest route to it is. And you are sometimes in a country where language is a big problem: it can be challenging even to find someone who can speak English.

The tour I went on this summer was hectic as usual. At least it was America. No language problems. Good facilities. We even got to base ourselves in the one place for two games running. Luxury! But it's still a bit annoying that the commercial and marketing departments dictate a club's pre-season schedule instead of concentrating on what is best for the players' preparation. In the old days the biggest issue during tours like this would be players drinking and getting into trouble and generally showing up for morning sessions a little the worse for wear. That culture is gone now so our main problem is dealing with the environmental changes that touring brings.

Salvation comes from the strangest places on tour. When Chelsea were in New York a few years back, when José Mourinho was the manager, one of their obligations was to do a photo shoot for their shirt sponsors, Samsung. They duly turned up, but when Mourinho found out that there was nothing in it for the players, he ordered them all to get back on the bus. Then suddenly, as if by magic, the latest plasma screen TVs started turning up on the players' doorsteps back home – and the natural order of things was restored . . .

The biggest problem of all about being on tour? I'm away from home when I don't want to be, and I'm working more as a roadie than a physio. When I return, people say, 'Well lucky you, that must have been brilliant!' These people also assume that because I am at a Premier League club I must be earning at least £50K a week but for some reason living the life of a tight git. Too mean to buy a Bentley!

As Donald Trump might say, so unfair.

We're fast approaching the end of August now, and we have played two games so far this season, with mixed results. Every-body seems pleased, but I don't see how we look any better than last season. I think most people are just pleased that the ship seems to be steady. The default mentality at some clubs is pes-simism bordering on panic. Even when things are going well people think it is just a reprieve from disaster. We're not quite like that. We enjoy success and we are envious of the clubs that have come out of the traps at top speed. Yet we have known enough bad periods that we can remind ourselves that even if things aren't perfect they have been worse.

The squad seems happy. This is part of the pathology of foot-ball clubs. When a manager departs, even if he wasn't loathed by the time he left there will certainly have been the smell of decay wafting from him for quite a while. So he gets the sack and people make the right noises and the media wonder if the poor man had a terminal case of 'losing the dressing room'. The obituaries often state that the players should 'have a good look at themselves'. Whether the dearly departed had suffered acute dressing-room loss or not, the arrival of his replacement puts all sorts of pressure on the players to perform for the new man. In romantic terms it's a way of saying to the ex-manager, 'Look, it wasn't us, it was you!'

So, early doors, everybody is chirpy and trying hard. A middling start to the season is interpreted as a good thing even if the games have been against teams that finished below us last season.

Thirty-six league games (plus a few cup runs) to go and no catastrophes have been presented to us in the medical room. But we do have a young centre-half recovering from the dreaded anterior cruciate ligament (ACL) injury. He has his career ahead of him. In his absence his reputation seems to grow. Reporters and fans seem unanimous that he will give us a greater range of options when he recovers. As such, he is a good patient. Happy, and good company. His view of his misfortune is simply that shit happens. He's right. He just takes this on as another challenge in his professional career and does everything he is asked to do. Good pro!

Our other long-term resident is a former captain, a frighteningly combative midfielder in his day. He's coming off a bad injury to his Achilles tendon which he has been a little impatient about. Who can blame him? He has many more games behind him than he has ahead of him. He has looked after himself well over the years and he has always been one of the more forceful personalities on and off the pitch.

The sad truth is that his injury is slow to heal, and that's a blessing. It's hard to see a place for his specialities within the sort of game we are playing. Being injured means he can rail against the misfortune of suffering a setback which is common to older players. He doesn't have to confront the fact that essentially it's all over for him. He should be making plans for the rest of his life. If he gets fit this season he might see some action in the League Cup and the early rounds of the FA Cup. He may go out and play a few games for the Under-23s. That's a sad way to finish a career.

There is an argument in favour of a player playing for as long as his body allows him to do so. For some players I agree with that, and my job is to make that happen for them. It's sad to see some guys on the fringes, though, overtaken and quickly forgotten by the fans who once sang their name in unison. I reckon our former captain isn't going to be match fit for another two months. Then it's going to get tough, unless he fancies a year or two in China making more money than he has made in his entire career so far.

It's transfer deadline day, and in the medical room we wait, listening to the news and expecting incoming like a M*A*S*H unit.

This is extra work we don't need. A normal pre-signing medical takes one or two days. It can take that long because it entails a full examination by the club doctor and/or physio, MRI scans and X-rays of their joints, heart screening, body composition testing and maybe even physical fitness testing. If the player has a long injury history it can take even longer as more specialist advice may be required. This is usually done without access to their medical records as the player has been rapidly transported to you and there hasn't been time to get hold of them.

In the past, I have been asked to do a medical with less than an hour to spare. Some of these last-minute deals are worth millions of pounds and there is simply no time for a more extensive medical.

After all the in-depth analysis of their current state of health, you provide the board with a report, usually verbal but backed up later in written form. You may get asked questions like 'Is the player fit then?' or 'Is that knee that has had three operations over the past two years and allowed him to play only ten games in two seasons going to hold up for a three-year contract?' Questions that only Derren Brown can answer with 100 per cent confidence.

I was once called to the chairman's office, with the manager, after completing a medical on an older player. I explained that the player had no anterior cruciate ligament intact and probably hadn't had one for a while. This meant that his knee could severely re-injure at any time. We do the tests in the knowledge that if the manager or chairman really, really wants to sign this guy because of his stats, or for whatever reason, it doesn't matter if we conclude after an hour or so that the player only has one functioning leg. If the club are desperate to sign him, they'll sign him regardless of what he might have wrong with him. I added that it was amazing that this guy had continued to play at all, but that he was a bit of a 'cart horse'. He could read the game incredibly well, so turning fast wasn't necessary.

After I'd presented all the facts, the chairman looked towards the manager and said, 'Well, do you feel lucky?'

The manager nodded. 'Yeah. I was born lucky.'

We signed the knackered player. Three-year deal.

He lasted six months. Science beat luck, as usual. The player broke down. Then the club continued to pay him £160K a week to sit around the treatment room. But by then everybody had forgotten the 'Do you feel lucky?' moment.

We have also heard of players who failed a medical at one club only to pass one at another. Demba Ba comes to mind. Spurs declined the risk. Chelsea signed him and managed it. They felt lucky and got lucky.

The two annual transfer deadline days are odd diversions from routine but not especially exciting or satisfying. If a player is presented to us in the afternoon of 31 August for a medical, while his entourage of agents, friends, parents and hangers-on wait around for the deal to be signed on the dotted line, we just do our best to be as thorough as we can with the caveat that time has allowed for only a cursory check compared to what we would like to do.

It is an ideal time, though, to take some baseline data from the player just in case we need it in the future. For example, by testing his knee ligaments or doing a scan we can find out what is 'normal' when he is fit so that if anything happens in the future we have a comparison. It is also a good time to start to build a relationship with the player. Joining a new club, often in a new country, is a very stressful time for players so a familiar face during their first few weeks can help them settle in.

Throughout August, managers go about mumbling their mantra. Have to make the squad stronger. Have to sign somebody. Anybody. Sometimes a club wants to sign a player and they just go with whatever specimen is presented to them. One of my favourite medical stories concerns Neil Ruddock, the sort of well-upholstered centre-half you just don't see any more.

When he joined West Ham in the summer of 1998 he was apparently asked to do a bleep test, the sort where you have to outrun the bleeps, which progressively get closer and closer together.

The physio said to Ruddock, 'Now this is the bleep test. I'm sure you've done it before. It's part of the medical.'

Ruddock looked at the physio in pure horror. 'You're having a fackin' laugh, mate. I thought this medical would just be asking me to lie down and wiggle things around a bit.'

'No, this is part of the medical exam I'm afraid.'

'Shit. What level do I have to get to?'

'Fourteen would be average.'

'Fourteen? Mate, I haven't done that since I was eight years old.'

I'm not sure if they took the precaution of having a defibrillator on hand but apparently he got to fourteen, or close enough, and then nearly dropped dead. But the box was ticked and West Ham signed him.

Usually, though, a medical provides only a snippet of info in that moment in time. Your intention is to pick up on the scary issues, such as cardiac problems. Many players have an enlarged heart as a result of years of being so fit and active. This can show up on screening as 'abnormal' and needs further investigation. The last thing you want is to put a player's life at risk. The sight of Marc-Vivien Foé collapsing on the field while playing for his country haunts me to this day.

Sometimes we talk to the manager and explain that the player he wants to sign has a physical issue but that we think we can manage it if he is used sensibly. It puts a bit of pressure on the medical room but that just makes the job interesting, and it's what we are paid for.

What makes transfer deadline days extra tricky is that you sometimes have no time to get information from the other club. You have to rely on the player to give you his own history. If he needs this transfer to get away from life as a sub or from a manager who hates him, or to be nearer to his roots or nearer to earning his third million, then it's not in his interest or his agent's to say to me, 'Oh by the way, you might like to double-check my right knee. I think it's knackered.' Sometimes you get medical records from a club and it looks as though someone has used the same pen to record all his details over the previous three years. In fact, judging by how hazy the information is, they probably wrote the whole three years' worth of records that morning.

A lot of clubs now make players sign a disclaimer so that if they give false information pertaining to the outcome of a medical the club has a fallback. As medics, we are protected too. So they need to be pretty honest with you, regardless of what the records show.

If there is a problem that the player or the selling club is worried about they will often do everything to delay the medical until as late as possible on transfer day. That ratchets up the pressure on everybody and means that the medical will be more hurried than we would like, and the buying club won't have the time to explore other options if a problem does arise.

Imagine the scene: it's nine in the evening on deadline day and you have to tell your harassed manager, who thinks that the player you are examining is the solution to all his problems, that said player seems to have a bum knee. He might get to the end of the season or he might break down next week. The manager will usually roll the dice and hope to get a few months out of the player. When the club is desperate to sign, all I can do is give the manager all the information I have available. It's that 'I feel lucky' moment again.

For a physio, a player's history is one of the most important things. A hamstring-prone player is at high risk of further such injuries; if he has got to the age of twenty-eight and not had a hamstring problem, the risk is low. I want to know how many games a player has played in the last three years. If I see he has only played twelve games in three years because of injuries, that tells me what his condition is going to be like for the next three years. The biggest indicator for injury is past injury. If he's only played twelve games simply because he's not been picked, that's different – but in that case I want training data. I want to know the reasons for the player not being fit. Minutes on the field is the most important indicator of how many minutes we can get out of the player.

A player with a recurring injury, or one that is likely to crop up again? That's a risk management decision. We just provide the information as best we can. After that it's up to the club as to what they do with that information.

I remember Arsenal signing the Swedish midfielder Kim Källström in the January 2014 transfer window. He was taken on with a back injury and wasn't available for more than four weeks. Apparently, he had managed to rick his back while playing volleyball on a beach in Abu Dhabi. (Now, who said a winter break was a good idea?) Despite Arsenal carrying out a 'medical' in order to screen the player for old and potential injuries, the club still signed Källström. Did they underestimate the extent of the injury at the time or did they not have enough time to interpret the implications of such an injury?

The medics were clearly rushed. The scan was done at five p.m. on the Friday, only hours before the transfer window closed, and it showed a small fracture in one of Källström's vertebrae. So why did the manager sanction the move, despite the Swede's previous club Spartak Moscow paying all his wages for the first six weeks? Arsène Wenger stated that, with the deadline approaching, he was forced into a decision as they were desperate to sign someone as cover for other injured and unavailable players in the same position. That sort of lame drum roll didn't exactly set Källström up to be a fan favourite. The Swede's career never really took off after that.

Back in 2012, Chelsea signed a player called Marko Marin who, it was said, was going to be the 'German Messi'. Which is probably why I took an interest. What would a German Messi be like? Individual, but in a very ordered way? A maverick who runs like clockwork? Anyway, Marin was signed with a hamstring injury and then didn't play for the Blues for three months. They had signed him on a five-year deal. As a physio you are thinking, 'Hey, what brain were you guys using? You've signed an injured player who has a history of hamstring problems!' I bet somebody felt lucky that day.

For the next five years Marin had hamstring issues. He ended up playing 143 minutes of league football for Chelsea. His loan spells with Sevilla, Fiorentina, Anderlecht and Trabzonspor were all punctuated by long periods in the physio room. The last three of those loan deals came with an option to buy but the state of the poor guy's hamstring meant he kept getting moved on before Olympiacos in Greece finally took him on a three-year deal.

Now Marin was once a German international and, along with Mesut Özil, part of a really good Werder Bremen team. Maybe he was worth a punt, but buying a player who comes with an injury like that is always a risk.

On the flip side, when a player is going to a club and is due for a medical he might come to me and say, 'Fucking hell, mate, how am I going to get through my medical with this knee?' I tell them what to say and what not to say in order to get through the process. The right information has to be given – they can't lie – but if they know *what* information to give they will usually get through. Three weeks later they will be having a knee operation, but that's the new club's problem for not asking the right questions.

Taking on a seasoned Premier League player with a history of significant injuries is a recipe for disaster. He will carry the two highest risk factors – age and injury history. Clubs are better off signing younger, injury-free players. The up-and-coming talents, particularly those who have coped with the 'natural selection' process of the academy system, are a start.

Also, lifestyle, family life, interests and personality are all enormously significant factors affecting how a player will fit into the squad and perform, as well as reliable indicators of how professional he will be and how hard he will work. Consequently, many teams are spending more and more time analysing the character of a player nowadays, not just videos of them playing.

It is even worth finding out how robust and tough they are: whether they are the sort that pull out at the hint of a niggling calf or shrug it off and carry on regardless. Usually a quick phone call to someone who knows the player will tell you what you need to know.

I remember the frustration of Harry Redknapp, then the Queens Park Rangers manager, over the voluptuous Adel Taarabt and how his lifestyle and weight issues apparently led to reduced performance and vulnerability to injury.

I hear of many teams doing hours in the gym in an attempt to prevent injury. Saliva samples are taken to monitor indicators for illness, and electronic devices are used to monitor heart-rate variability for signs of stress and fatigue. For me, the essentials stay the same. Have a great coach who knows how to prepare a team psychologically and physically for games. Sleep well – still the best recovery strategy out there. Eat well: steer clear of processed foods, and try to go organic (not too much pasta, though). Minimize alcohol. Hydrate efficiently. And be fit to play football the way you play your football. What is physically right for the centre-half is not always right for the winger. (I think that's from the Bible.) Do those things and you won't be looking back with tears in your eyes at a succession of transfer deadline day duds. You won't have media asking you about 'where it all went wrong with the dream move'.

As it turns out, today is mercifully quiet as deadline days go. We do three medicals. The first player leaves, gets into his Jeep with his agent and skedaddles. We hear later in the day that he has signed a contract elsewhere. In the afternoon we sign two young players, both healthy specimens and both likely to vanish on loan deals before we really get to know them. We then hear on Sky that the club has concluded its business for the day.

Well, that was easy. Let's go home then.

TSF: Second Opinion

Medicals

Medicals are anomalies. They're like black holes in space. They don't fit the model of modern medical practice. They result in outcomes that are inexplicable.

If a manager really wants a player then he will tell the club doctor to overlook the odd injury from yesteryear, even the odd piece of shrapnel. José Mourinho, for instance, had such a hard-on for Paul Pogba that I imagine if left to his own devices he would have signed the Frenchman even if he had been on life support. Mourinho needed him as a trophy signing; he needed to pay a record sum of money to show everybody that he had the size of cojones necessary to manage at Old Trafford. Even better, it was a record wad splashed on a player whom Fergie had once rejected.

For the doctors at United that would have been a tough one to deal with. Rock and a hard place springs to mind. There was so much money at stake. Pogba's agent was getting more than most players will ever move for. No medical pro could have lowered the bar for Pogba. It's the medics who sign off on these deals at the end of the day. Still, they must have felt the heat of

Mourinho's ardour and fretted about being caught in the cross-fire if anything went wrong.

My favourite example is when Stoke's manager at the time, Tony Pulis, was so desperate to sign Peter Crouch that the canny Tottenham chief executive Daniel Levy managed to persuade Pulis to take Wilson Palacios too. Thirteen million all in, Tone. Take it or leave it.

Palacios, as everybody in the game knew, had a degenerative knee complaint which meant that he only played once in a blue moon, or thirty-eight times in four years, whichever figure was medically advisable. Crouchy is a bit willowy but as indestructible as a Panzer tank by comparison.

When you own a club and appoint your manager, you pays your money and takes your chances. Or chancers.

My own medicals were a joke. When I signed for my first league side from my non-league club, the shysters involved in the deal were so desperate for the £1,500 'drink' they'd been promised that no club doctor was going to get in their way. Doctors' opinions were dismissed as breezily as economics experts in the Brexit debate.

He'll be fucking fine.

When I was transferred to my first big club, the same shysters were still on the take, so the deal went through smoothly. It had to. I touched my toes, wiggled my dodgy ankle, and lo and behold I was given a clean bill of health and pronounced fitter than a Navy SEAL.

When I moved for countless millions to a big Premier League club there was of course a feeding frenzy for my services. Whatever. The same set of fundamentally bendy laws played out.

He'll do. We'll get a couple of years out of him with regular servicing.

On it went, right to the end of my career when I became a 'named' signing with smaller clubs. By 'named' I mean that when people googled me they turned to each other and said, 'Yeah, it's that twat all right.'

Despite all my injuries, I had just enough credibility as a saviour for the club doctor to ignore all of my physiological problems. And that's generally the norm in football. They want your body, not your sunny personality.

Dick Dastardly

There is nothing sadder than a physio who is controlled by an overbearing manager. The manager generally remembers how things were done back in the day when men were men etc. and missing a game because your leg was hanging off meant that you were a namby-pamby fanny who might have a touch of Johnny Foreigner blood in his veins.

From a player's point of view, the best physios are the ones whom the manager absolutely trusts. If the physio says that the player needs a few days in the sun or a day off or a day in the pool instead of the gym, then that's what he needs. No argument.

Those managers who don't trust their physios any more than they trust their players tend to want to interfere with rehab. They are racked by a Trumpian paranoia and think that everybody at their own club is out to get them.

I have played for such creatures. The truth is that when you are injured you actually work harder and longer than anybody else at the club because you're in at nine a.m. and away by five, as opposed to the playing squad who are in at ten a.m. and home by one most days.

Being injured is exhausting and draining, lonely and depressing. Good physios spot when an injured player just needs to take some time out. They know when a change is as good as a rest, and vice versa. I'm talking about long-term injuries here, not injuries where the player is out for a week or two. The best physio I ever worked with used to say, 'Sometimes a rest is better than a run.' And it's absolutely true. I would go so far as to say 'A rest is always better than a run', but that's a layman's view.

When I round off my bucket list with the names of the people I want to have bumped off by contract killers, a certain manager I once played under will be sure to appear. Let's call him Dick Dastardly.

One day Dick Dastardly picked a team to play Liverpool, and to everybody's surprise he included me in the line-up. I'd been in rehab all morning and every morning for the previous three months before that with another knee injury.

He didn't tell me or the physio that he was going to pick me. Surprise!

I remember when he flipped over the A-board in the dressing room and my name was on the team sheet. Fuck me.

The lads just stared at me with wry smiles on their faces. I realized what the manager was doing. He hated me and he had me by the balls. He was digging a hole, picking me to lie in it, and then he would shovel the dirt down on top of me.

I was just about fit enough to go on the pitch but definitely not fit enough to do myself any justice. Worse, if I said that I wasn't going to risk myself by playing he would get all leaky with the media and let it be known that I was refusing to play. I'd be the cad and bounder letting the club, his team-mates and the whole city down. At the time he was putting an awful lot of pressure on me to leave. He put me in a real catch-22 position where I had to play and underperform or refuse to play and get slated.

We managed to steal a draw in what was one of the most awful football matches in the history of the game. I fitted right in and survived for another while at least.

Holding back the swell

Physios handle Voltarol like drunks handle confetti at a wedding. They chuck them about with an air of abandon and nobody worries about the mess. You see, Voltarol solves everything from dodgy knees to the heartache of marital breakdown.

Voltarol is an anti-inflammatory pill that stops bleeding in the muscles. Bleeding in the muscles happens after every single workout. If you lift weights then your muscles break apart, and then they repair themselves by knitting back together again and becoming stronger. That's how muscle is grown on top of muscle.

Footballers don't want to become too heavy in terms of muscle because they need to be agile. (No, really.) So they chomp Voltarol. Voltarol allows players to strengthen their bodies but stops the pesky bleeding in the muscles that would lay down new muscle and lead to them becoming too big to play – a condition known as Ruddockitis. Stop the bleeding and you largely stop new muscle growth. You cut off the supply of blood to new muscle. Smart, or cheating?

(And yes I am being paid extra for the number of times I can use the word 'muscle' in one paragraph. Times are hard.)

Voltarol isn't illegal in football because it has a legitimate use for injuries. It can retard the effects of a dead leg or a badly bruised bone, the sort of injuries that could keep a player out for one or two games. Easily remedied with a magic tablet. And because of that, like so many legitimate drugs, it has been abused for its additional benefits.

If you want a tip from a pro, take Voltarol before you go out drinking (but always follow the instructions, folks). Its anti-inflammatory properties stop the brain from swelling, and swelling of the brain is the leading cause (apart from alcohol) of all hangovers. At our Christmas parties, the physio would hand out packets of Voltarol before we boldly went where so many professionals had very boldly gone before. This still goes on. And why not? It's a no-brainer, so to speak.

So if you're going out this weekend, take Voltarol before you go, and then swig down a glass of water between every alcoholic drink. You will never have another hangover ever again. That, kids, is sensible drinking.

A swell time

I can recall injuring my knee pretty badly in one particular match and hobbling off to the physio room while the game was still going on.

Our physio room at that time had a big 42-inch plasma TV in it. It was tuned to Jeff Stelling, who brought us all the scores from around the country in his usual enthusiastic style.

We were ignoring that, and the shouts and moans of distress filtering into the physio room from the tens of thousands of fans watching our game outside. Nobody quite knew how bad my knee was but we did know that it was a ligament injury because when the physio tested the knee to see if it would spring back, it didn't. I wasn't angry with my flaccid knee, just disappointed.

In fact when the physio tested the knee it offered no resistance at all, it simply kept going, as if it would be more comfortable and easy to store if folded in two. Classic signs that a ligament or two had ruptured.

If it was a medial ligament then the knee would swell up on the side – a good sign. But if it was a cruciate injury, the worst-case scenario, the whole knee wouldn't swell for a few hours.

Jeff Stelling was going mad at one end of the room, the crowd outside were baying for blood, and I had the feeling that I wasn't quite the centre of the universe as I, the physio, the club doctor and the tunnel steward, who'd wandered in for a nosey, sat in total silence staring at my traitorous knee.

After ten minutes it began to swell on the inside, indicating a medial ligament injury and not a cruciate. It was still a three-month lay-off but it also prompted the loudest cheer of the day – in my head anyway.

Unbelievable, Jeff.

SEPTEMBER

I'm not one for saying I told you so. But I told you so. Are we already seeing signs of burnout and higher injury rates with players who played in the Euros? I think so, and we have played only four games. It's not even mid-September yet!

We played twice this week. For the next three weeks we have games every three to four days. There are Premier League fixtures interspersed with games in Europe and the League Cup. We had it easy for the first three games of the season as they were only one a week. Now the hard work is beginning.

Not only do you have players who were on international duty all summer, but looking ahead they won't even get any respite when the league games ease up. They'll be called away for international weeks. I believe that playing matches is the best way to condition but rest is important both physically and mentally. At some stage the player needs to get off the hamster wheel.

The key is to manage a player's schedule, balancing game play – domestic and international – with appropriate levels of training and adequate rest periods. These days it takes a good three days to fully recover from a game. That's why anyone playing on a Saturday will next play on Tuesday at the earliest. Or if they play on a Sunday, they'll play next on the Wednesday.

Years ago, teams sometimes played on consecutive days, but the game is different now: it is faster, more intensive, more demanding. In 1972, Leeds famously won the FA Cup at Wembley on Saturday and lost the league away to Wolves on Monday night. And that was a long, long time before we had invented squad rotation.

The need for a recovery day the day after a game has been recognized for many years. The squad may do either a pool or bike session or ideally, on the field, carry out light-recovery jogging and stretching for forty-five minutes or so. But with the intensity of the game now, where players cover over 12km during a match, they need a second day of light-intensity work for forty-five to sixty minutes in order to avoid injury and fatigue in the next fixture.

We have a big squad and are happy with our level of player availability. There is a difference, though, between providing the manager with bodies fit enough to play and those bodies being at the peak of their fitness.

We shall see.

A lot of time in early season is spent just updating our stats. Glamour? You don't know the meaning of the word.

People imagine that physios spend all their time shining the legs of millionaire players and indulging in a bit of banter. Wrong! But I would say that wouldn't I? We see ourselves as cutting-edge scientists pushing the envelope year after year to make the world a better place. Until we get our pay cheque, that is.

Stats and data are an increasingly important part of our lives though. It is a necessary evil, though it always amazes me how little depth we add to our knowledge through statistics and data. If we could all share information we would have a better idea of when players get injured, why, what the ideal training load is, what injuries follow different managers around, etc. Everybody would win. But everybody winning isn't the point of football. In football we believe that it's better for your neighbour's horse to die than for you to have two horses.

The biggest influence on injury prevention is the coaches. They plan the intensity, content, volume and duration of each training session, and how it fits into the week, the month, the season. You don't get fit for a marathon by playing squash, and vice versa. To get fit to play football, you play football. The golden ticket is what you do in the days between games in order to prepare the player's body optimally for the next game. Many teams use GPS monitoring to work out a player's workload and come up with enormous amounts of data and algorithms calculating what targets the player must reach in order to be fit for the game. For me, this is a still unproven science and needs to be used with caution. It should only be used as a guide, not as the be-all-and-end-all of how you train.

The biggest problem is that no longitudinal season-by-season data has been collated to show what is best for each individual player in terms of preparation for a game. We are too proprietorial about the knowledge we accumulate. Squads change, players change, year in, year out – therefore, so does the data. In fact the 'average' data changes at every transfer window so comparisons should be drawn among individuals only, not on a team basis: for example, you would need to compare this year's Eden Hazard with last year's Eden Hazard. This process takes years. Then the manager and coach change, so the whole thing shifts again, and the data gets muddier.

Eden Hazard is a different animal from Mesut Özil who is different from Wayne Rooney who is different from Theo Walcott. Training has to be specific to a player's position, fitness and age. Yet we judge them all by the same criteria. One year Hazard is a waste of space. The next year it's Özil. Why can't he be more like Hazard? they ask.

In the medical room we operate just like any medical system out in the real world. We have to keep records. That protects the player, allows clubs that might buy him access to a detailed medical history, and it protects us in case anybody ever comes at us brandishing a barrister. These days we have computerized medical records which encapsulate everything. Match minutes, training minutes, even the specifics of what the training is. You log injuries, what happened, what you found on assessment, info from appointments with consultants, day-to-day treatment details, etc. You can do that using an iPhone which will download it on to a server. You can enter details of an injury while you are travelling back from a game on the bus.

I keep details on how much every player has played, how much they haven't, and when they have had a recurring problem. With that info we can anticipate when that problem might happen again in the future. I also like to build a picture of the workloads and mileage that each player can handle and what the needs are for players in specific positions.

There are two very important figures for teams. Match availability is the first – what percentage of the first-team squad is available to play for games. If we have 100 per cent match availability then every player is available for every game. That's impossible of course, because it would mean no injuries, illnesses, international duty, or wives going into labour. If you get over 90 per cent, that's good; over 95 per cent is incredibly good. That is the target. We track training availability too, though it doesn't really matter at the bottom line if a player is available to train. Matches are what is important. It is just common sense that if they miss a lot of training they will invariably get injured in games as they haven't done the correct amount of conditioning to be fit.

The other big measure of our department is a squad's re-injury rate. If you have had lots of players back in training who broke down again and again with the same injury, it's a poor reflection on us. You are not doing your job properly. (I should note that re-injuries are to be expected, though. If you are pushing the levels of performance and encouraging players to return asap, sometimes the odd player will break.)

We had a bad year last year.

There is a direct correlation between having good match availability stats and winning. The thing you find at the higher levels of the Champions League is that successful teams keep their player match availability high. The top teams simply get fewer injuries. I even think top players get injured less. It's a process of natural selection. Survival of the fittest and the best.

If our new manager has his best players available we will see less of him haunting the medical room, wondering when exactly the miracle healing will begin. He's a good guy but we don't want to bring him bad news too often or have him coming in here when he is stressed out and wondering if the centre-half can play on one leg this Saturday.

At training today the reserve right-winger went over on his ankle. He limped off, and I threw his arm around my shoulder and helped him to the medical room. I hadn't seen the incident but he let out a noise at the time which suggested he might have done damage.

Yet when we got to the medical room he sat on one of the beds and immediately announced that he was ready to go back out to training. We insisted that he needed to be looked at. There might be nothing to worry about but equally there might be an injury. Letting us look at it was the only professional option. He was very resistant to the idea.

The doc and I glanced at each other: we knew why. I don't have the stats on this, but I believe it to be true: a player's pain threshold improves when his contract is due to come up for negotiation. This is when the boy suddenly develops an amazing capacity to cope. If he wants to play badly enough he will find the will to go through walls.

Our winger is twenty-two. He doesn't get into the first team too often but he's rated highly enough that the club keeps him around instead of putting him on loan. His contract is up soon and he wants to stay here. He can't afford to be tucked away out of sight and out of mind in the medical room.

Some players, maybe in year two of a long contract, on the other hand, have such a low pain tolerance that I don't know how they even get out of bed in the morning. What amazes me is how those players have even reached the level they have got to.

I suppose the great thing about the academy system is the natural selection process. The system works out who is robust enough to play professional football. If you aren't strong enough you will break as a youth player. I look at some players who are in their peak playing years (at twenty-six or twenty-seven) and I am amazed that they have never picked up an injury. Either they are indestructible, like Suárez or John Terry, or they are incredibly talented and somebody will always buy them. Jack Wilshere. Daniel Sturridge. It's a battlefield out there. You may see them as an overpaid, whinging bunch of fannies but for professional footballers, pain is normal. If you can't train and play through pain you won't reach that top few per cent.

The low-pain-threshold guys are usually hugely talented and clubs have always taken a punt on them. Take Abou Diaby. Played 125 times for Arsenal. Not bad. But that was over nine years. That's an average of fourteen games per year. I think it was a low pain threshold but it could just have been bad luck.

Perhaps teams should take a 'Moneyball' approach, by which I mean spend some time comparing match minutes or availability with the amount of time a player is injured; they may get more value for money. They could also try incentivizing them to stay fit and therefore negate bad luck.

Football is very different from sports like cycling and athletics, which operate at the limit of physiological capability. Footballers rely a lot on talent. At my level I see top Prem players who are there solely because they are incredibly gifted. They could be even better if they took their physiology to another level.

They could be more athletic, stronger, faster. But usually they aren't that interested. That is the difference between the Ronaldos of this world and the decent Premier League players. Ronaldo squeezes *everything* out of his body.

Of course all footballers are there because they are talented to some degree. I've worked with bang average players who maximized their physical capability and made a living. I've worked with very good players who have been terrible athletes; had they been better athletes they could have played for a team like Manchester United. I get frustrated when I see those players: either they have not been encouraged, motivated or educated in self-improvement, or the club staff don't take the initiative to enlighten the players about fitness.

At bigger clubs some of the staff tend to be in awe of the players and let them do what they like. The Ferguson era at Old Trafford was different. Those players were pushed and pushed to be better – that's why they were successful – and that made it easier to push the next generation.

Behind every great man there is a woman. I'm not sure what there is behind every great woman. Probably another great woman, but one with a score to settle. In the medical room we like to think that behind every great football team there is a great medical team. But why are so few of the medical teams, great or otherwise, staffed with women? In other words, was Eva Carneiro an outlier?

It's September 2016, just over a year on from the Eva Carneiro affair. It seems longer somehow, as football moves along so fast. At this time of year I usually get letters from those students who want to come to the club to do placements or internships as physios. One thing that has always made me curious is why the female applicants usually include photos of themselves and the males almost never do.

In the Eva Carneiro case, she and the physio, Jon Fearn, were called on to the pitch by the referee to tend to Eden Hazard. There was no basis for them refusing to go on or to ask Chelsea manager José Mourinho's permission to do so. A player was requesting medical attention and the referee summoned them on. They did the right thing by going on. What should they have done? Refused to go on because Chelsea only had ten men (one had been sent off) on the field, and momentarily they would be down to nine players, and just hope Hazard was OK?

Mourinho was unprofessional in abusing them both as they came off the field and he was unprofessional in criticizing them publicly afterwards.

Unfortunately, working in football and expecting not to be abused from time to time is like working in a coal mine and hoping not to get your clothes dirty. I get abused and shouted at all the time. Managers and players are highly stressed people. You take it on the chin and do your job and forget about it.

Doesn't mean it's right though.

The result is not as important as the health of a player. Neither are your feelings. That is your stance as a medic. Obviously it isn't always the club's stance. And it's almost never the manager's stance.

Mourinho didn't criticize Hazard for staying down. He didn't even have a go at the referee for calling the medics on. He picked on the medics. That's the law of the jungle. Live with it. Rough with the smooth. Shit flows down the hill. Some days the manager abuses you, some days he apologizes to you (rarely though), some days he celebrates with you, and some days he thanks you.

That game between Chelsea and Swansea ended in a 2-2 draw. Had Chelsea scored a late winner after the incident the entire business would have been forgotten about.

Either way, the medical department's job is to get on with things. Physios and doctors have to make these decisions regularly. Yes, we may get it wrong occasionally. We all make mistakes.

Mourinho made a mistake. He behaved badly. Eva Carneiro lost a lot of sympathy in the game though when she went on social media about the issue, and later went to court and got a massive pay-off. Good for Eva Carneiro, but good for women in football?

The feeling in football was that if 'she' had been a 'he' there would never have been a fiasco (or enormous pay-off). Football is more old school in its prejudices and quietly sexist than a lot of other sports and it will only change through massive re-education and positive experiences.

Whatever the rights and wrongs of the Carneiro business it certainly dragged our trade kicking and screaming into the spotlight.

I worked at a club once where the manager insisted on employing a female physio purely because she 'had a nice arse', the glory of which he liked to survey from the touchline as she treated players. Never mind her rear end, her head certainly got turned and she got through dalliances with about half the team in the course of a season with us. That of course was her business, but when it grew into a problem within the squad it became the club's business. You can imagine the outcome.

Football is not a politically correct place. You might wish it to be but players are thrown into an all-male macho environment right from their early teens. Female influence is minuscule compared to the peer pressure exerted during a lifetime in football dressing rooms. If you travel with players you witness what little they have been taught in their young lives about feminism and respect being eroded very quickly by the battalions of groupies and wannabe WAGs who throw themselves at footballers.

So clubs often disregard the qualifications and abilities of female medics not out of pure sexism (though I am sure that exists) but because they understand the imperfect environment that is football and don't wish to complicate things further. They just won't take the risk. The success of the first team is the only issue that matters at a football club.

Back in 2003, a female physio at Crystal Palace sued the club after she had been selected for possible redundancy as part of a drive to cut costs. She was asked to take a pay cut or accept a redundancy package. She claimed at tribunal that the club's first-team physiotherapist should also have been put at risk of being let go because he had the same qualifications and similar experience to herself. Most ancillary staff at a football club have trouble with the notion that they can be asked to accept pay cuts or redundancies when first-team players are earning ever more obscene amounts, but that comes with the territory.

I have no reason to think that the female physio was anything other than a highly competent professional. That is surely how she achieved so much in our male-dominated profession. But she lost her case because Palace argued that the first-team physio was just that, the first-team physio. The first team matters most. They didn't want change to occur there. In the world of football, everything comes second to winning.

It's right that from time to time somebody should hold the feet of a football club's directors to the fire if they feel they have a grievance, but clubs don't enjoy the process and I'm pretty sure the overall effect of cases involving women is that clubs quietly shy away from employing female professionals, in the medical room and elsewhere.

Players have changed and the medical staff have changed but nobody who works in football walks around with a directory of labour laws in their pocket. You expect to work long, irregular hours and you expect that you will be shouted at and occasionally bullied by managers who are under pressure or by players who are stressed. Managers often shout the same question at physios: 'Who do you work for? Tell me who you think you work for!' The answer they want to hear is, 'You. I work for you.'

It's the same with chairmen or owners. They want to hear you say that you work for them.

My policy is to tell them whatever they want to hear. Yeah, I work for you. There are no politics involved in it for me. No greasy pole that I have to climb to get to the boardroom or wherever. I just want peace and the space in which to work for the people I really work for – the players. It doesn't matter who pays my wages or how desperately the manager needs to have a patched-up centre-half play ninety minutes in twenty-four hours' time, the duty of care is to the patient. Anything else is malpractice. So I just do my job and don't comment.

'I envy you your job, mate. The places you get to see. The excitement. It's like your life is a paid holiday.'

The man standing beside me at the school gate doesn't know it but he has just moved on to what I recognize as part two of the standard chat when someone finds out you are a football physio. Part one is their disbelief at who you work for – 'Really? Nah, you're taking the piss, mate' – followed by the question, 'What's so-and-so like? . . . Nah, what's he *really* like?'

The conversation then moves on with your new friend telling you how you have the greatest job in the world.

'Do you get to see all the games?'

'Yeah.'

'Are you one of the blokes who runs on to the pitch?'

'Yeah.'

'I tell you something, mate.'

'What?'

'I really do envy you your job . . .'

Really? There I stand, remembering working at Colchester on a cold Tuesday night in January, strapping an ankle in the shower as water dripped on the back of my head. Every time I moved, a new source of water would find me. Or Rotherham, where in the old stadium they had a sauna in the dressing room. It always seemed to be on. I shed pounds in that dressing room.

I think about those grounds where you had to manoeuvre skips full of medical gear down steps or up steps, wrestling with them like removal men with a baby grand – like at good old Highbury.

At some grounds they would wet the floor of the away team dressing room. You take your boot off. Foot is wet. The wetness starts niggling at the back of your head. The manager is speaking his words of wisdom and you are looking around the room trying not to shout something about the dangers of verrucas and trench foot.

Fulham's changing room is so small there's not enough space to set the kit up. Wigan share their space with the rugby league team, and the room is so massive that you just can't see where the manager is. The first-team dressing room at the Emirates is all feng shui curves; the away-team dressing room is all boxes and squares and corners. Staff in one room, players somewhere else.

Purple walls at Chelsea for the away team! Prince would have loved playing there, but it really was depressing. They had decided that this was the worst colour for a dressing room. They were right. It did your head in.

Then there's the logistical headache of trying to get things set up so that you can give adequate attention to the players who need it. We need to have at least four beds, but at some grounds you're lucky if you can squeeze two into the dressing room. You might end up working in a corridor or in the shower area. Highbury was notoriously bad for this. You had to put beds in the shower, and the floor was angled so you had to make a strategic decision as to which way you wanted the bed to tilt.

At Manchester City, the first-team dressing room is a palace but the away team gets changed in an area with a slanted roof that is almost like a corridor. It is one of the nice ones though because at least there is space. Players hate sitting with players on either side of them in their personal space. They like to have cubicles with wood frames which delineate their own space.

Generally, though, players just want to get out of the dressing room and on to the pitch. And nowhere is it better to do that than in the stadiums of continental Europe. The noise – it hits you like something physical, something elemental. The din is incredible at some games, a form of electricity. That's what big European games mean to me – the Italian teams, or grounds in the Ukraine or Istanbul. The noise just comes right down and hits you over the head. In England you don't feel it, although Anfield before a game starts comes close. I always remember a quote from John Terry talking about how the hairs on the back of his neck stand up when the Kop breaks into 'You'll Never Walk Alone'. I have to agree.

Italian stadiums are like being at a nightclub and sitting beside the speaker. Your ears crackle. At some games my ears are crackling the whole time from kick-off to final whistle. My nerves jangle. For a player it must be awe-inspiring just as much as it is intimidating.

I think of those nights and, yeah, it *is* a great job.

We are lucky to be in Europe this year. It's a lot of travel and work but those nights in those places? The noise and the gladiators?

OK, I'm envious of myself sometimes.

One thing I found as a result of the Eva Carneiro circus was that it caused a spike in the number of people asking me if players are really injured when I run on to the pitch – or are their injuries 'fake news'? And how do I know if it is serious? Is it annoying to be seen running on for a potentially serious issue only to find out that there is nothing wrong?

The most important factor here is to know your players. You have to know the ones who go down easily. With these, I hesitate before sprinting on to the pitch and invariably, given a bit of time, a miracle occurs and they are fine. Many times I have run on to the pitch, asked the player what is wrong and heard the gasped whisper: 'I'm fine, just need a minute. I'm knackered.'

That's when we go through the motions of 'faking' an injury. It's quite creative really. The odd time I have left a player on his back moving his legs as if slowly riding a bicycle. I walk over to the fourth official and just abandon the 'cyclist' there in front of 50,000 fans.

And yes, I have been involved in staging some of these collaborative productions just before international breaks in order for the player to avoid going away with his country. Somebody should do a study of the number of top players who pick up minor knocks just before pointless international friendlies. If those friendlies are away from home or in another continent the problem gets even worse.

By the way, leaving a player on the touchline doing a slow bicycle movement so that he then has to stand up and brush himself down and tell the fourth official that he can resume at the next break of play is just payback. Some referees kill me by calling me on to the pitch too soon, without checking with the player. I get halfway there and the player runs away!

As soon as I step on to the field to assess a player, he has to come off until the game restarts. So if I am called on when we have just conceded a corner in the 89th minute and we are 1-0 up, and the player I'm called on for is a strong centre-half who is intending to mark their big centre-forward . . . you can see the dilemma.

How do I know it's serious? Sometimes it's just obvious if you have seen the incident that caused the injury and you muttered the words 'Oh shit'.

Sometimes it's the player. When a player who you know can carry a strong tackle and who normally jumps up after an incident stays down or takes longer to get moving again, or the situation just looks serious – i.e. the player isn't moving, or we've all heard a loud crack – then I spring into action.

Thankfully, serious incidents are not that common. The number of times I run on to the pitch and the player is safe continues to far outweigh the times when I have to remove the player from the field with a serious injury.

As for gamesmanship . . . is that coffee you smell as you wake up? This is professional football! It is completely understandable that players maximize every possible situation to gain an advantage over the opposition, and being tackled is no exception. It would be naive to think otherwise. I realize that it has got worse with the minor contacts, or no contact at all, but sometimes the sanctimony of former players now working as pundits and feigning horror about these things makes me want to put a few highlight reels together of their own best performances in the categories of diving and writhing around.

Lastly, I have never heard of a manager or coach telling a player to go down easily and I've never seen it practised on the training ground. That suggestion is ridiculous. I have seen many players get hurt in training during tackles, so the idea of theatrically rehearsing going to ground to simulate a tackle scenario is just madness.

I've often had players coming to look for treatment that I don't really believe they will benefit from. Maybe they want acupuncture. Their mate will have had acupuncture and reckoned it was the dog's doodahs so now they want acupuncture too. Or maybe they want to work on that machine over there.

'I want that machine.'

'Why?'

'I really think it will help.'

'You do know what it's for, don't you?'

'Ehm . . .'

If they believe in something and it isn't detrimental to them I'll just tell them to go right ahead. One of the best treatments you can have is a placebo treatment. If the player has faith in it and thinks that the treatment is powerful, well, I'll let him have it. Many players have gone on to see 'gurus' who have been recommended to them by fellow pros. In reality, going to see someone outside the club, in a nice private clinic, is automatically going to have a positive placebo effect. The guru performs some weird unfamiliar technique or lays on some bullshit about how effective this treatment is and the player is sold on it. I'm not always convinced, and I have seen a few.

But I'm fascinated by placebos and how they work on our minds. The colour, shape, taste and even name of a simple tablet actually has an impact on how effective that medication will be. It was summed up in an unlikely way in an article in *The Atlantic* a few years ago. The American magazine pointed out that in the TV series *Breaking Bad*, Walter White's business soon 'becomes all about the blue – from drug addicts to rival producers, everyone wants White's signature tint'. The fictional meth manufacturer isn't the only one who understands the importance of drug colour. On both sides of the law, it's a key part of branding. Viagra is famously known as 'the little blue pill', Nexium is marketed as 'the purple pill', and street names for illicit drugs run through the whole rainbow.

The placebo effect of drugs is heightened by their colour. We tend to associate colours with specific effects. Blue pills act best as sedatives, except – and I swear that there is research on this – on Italian males who associate the colour with the Azzurri and the excitement of football. Red and orange are stimulants. Green calms us, and white makes pain go away. Bright yellow is a good sunny colour for antidepressants. 'A bright yellow pill,' *The Atlantic* article noted, 'with the name on its surface, for example, may have a stronger effect than a dull yellow pill without it.'

It's not ethical sometimes to give a player an anti-inflammatory just because they demand it but sometimes a player adamantly insists that he wants one. You know it isn't going to do him any good and it might actually be detrimental to his recovery. It doesn't help to stamp your foot and say, 'No, I have my ethics and I don't really care if your last club handed out anti-inflammatories like Smarties, I'm not giving you one.' But if you give them something harmless and let them think it's an anti-inflam? You're winning. There is an ethical issue in that

I'm not giving them the tablet they think they are getting, but then placebos can be up to 60 per cent effective.

Likewise, if a player believes that sticking an ultrasound on his quad will make it better then I'll do it. Ultrasound on a quad is a complete waste of time. The muscle is too thick and bloody. The ultrasound gets dispersed rather than absorbed. But hey, if the player is happy . . .

Ultrasound is a ubiquitous bit of kit these days. A smaller club may not have laser, which costs tens of thousands, or a shockwave machine, which is also tens of thousands. But everybody has ultrasound.

What is amazing is that recovery rates remain basically the same. Most players will have come across ultrasound machines on their way up the ladder and will have faith in them. So if the manager wants a player back at training in two days' time the placebo treatment of the ultrasound may get him over the line. You are working on the marginal gains. Like Team Sky but in a healthier general environment.

The small percentages matter. Create an environment where every little thing is worked on and you are doing your best. You accumulate anecdotal evidence based on experience, research, your own experiences and the players' preferences as to what they like and what their rehab cultures and beliefs are. You throw all that into your clinical reasoning and conclude that anything that may help and has no risk attached to it should be considered.

And if you have to dupe them with the odd placebo, just remember Walter White and his blue meth.

TSF: Second Opinion

Yoga for the masses

When yoga and meditation became all the rage, every club had to have a visiting guru or yogi come in every week – otherwise relegation was inevitable. My Premier League club humoured us by hiring a beautiful and very friendly blonde woman who could stretch herself into unlikely positions for our gratification. We would gather and watch and think impure thoughts.

She would sit, all serene and lovely and spread out, in front of twenty-five of us rapt students, who had fought like dogs for a spot on the mat that was laid out immediately in front of her. For a while she was the best part of the week.

However, the lessons soon became a source of tension among us. Some of the less committed yoga novices reckoned that having seen her stretch two or three times they didn't need to see her stretch any more, unless she was going to add some lascivious twerking to the routine.

Numbers dropped off. The yoga crisis deepened when some players began to get arsey with each other because it appeared as if she had guru's pets. She'd show special attention to one player as he smirkingly pretended to struggle with his downward-facing dog. The rest of us achieved oneness with our green-eyed jealousy.

(I tried to lighten the mood with the old joke about the Dalai Lama ordering at the hotdog stand. Make me one with everything. Not the right audience. Dalai ding, Dalai dong.)

Eventually our manager had to let the lithe guru go. He

claimed that we hadn't really embraced the idea of yoga. We were more interested in the messenger than the message. The gains he had hoped we would make had never really materialized. He would remain disappointed in us, for this life anyway.

Her departure didn't bring harmony to the squad, however. Freed from the need to keep a professional distance, she began dating her way through the squad. Thankfully the players involved were far too mature and enlightened to compare notes on the various and surprising positions the guru could adopt in more private settings.

That would have just been bad karma.

Pranker

As clubs become bigger deals to a whole range of people, they attract blizzards of requests from ambitious student types looking to gain work experience with Championship and Premier League outfits.

One physio I worked with was genuinely very keen to offer this experience to the next generation of leg shiners and muscle tweakers, but he also recognized that a spare pair of hands with the massages and menial tasks would be a very welcome short-term dividend of his altruism.

Some of these graduates were fine, but others had unfeasibly large rods up their arses. They were looking to buff their self-importance by attaching the name of a Premier League football club to their CV. The act of having successfully plugged in an ultrasound machine one morning would later appear on the CV as having 'worked closely with Luis Suárez and Steven

Gerrard through diagnosis and rehab at critical parts of a highly pressurized season'.

So it became necessary to tamper with the mental well-being of these particular upstarts. Harmless japes included stealing the keys to one of their battered cars and re-parking the vehicle in the middle of the training pitch on the centre circle before the manager arrived. The entire medical room would shake their heads in a unified display of sanctimony and despair as the gaffer bawled out the baffled kid.

Tut. What *were* you thinking, son? The gaffer hates you now.

The placement kid would make the rookie mistake of protesting his innocence and announcing, perhaps, that his father's business partner once worked for Amnesty International and this shit was worse than waterboarding – like seriously, dudes, not funny.

Some of them took it better than that and went up in our estimation. Others let their eyes well up and announced that they were not cut out for a life in football. We felt as if we were separating the wheat from the chaff and that future generations would benefit from our work.

Other educational innovations included wittily writing words like 'Clueless' or 'Loser' on the bottom of an intern's coffee mug and then asking the boys who ran the website to interview him on camera to see how he was getting on and make sure they captured him raising his mug to his lips. They'd quickly edit it and then post it online and the comedy classic would immediately go viral in the dressing room.

Once we went too far though. We had a young lady in for the week and, annoyingly, she was actually very nice and genuinely keen to get on in the game. She wouldn't have made it as a physio at the top level because, as they might say in Newcastle, she was reet petite and just didn't have the physique. That was her problem, not ours, and we didn't let her frailty or her gender interfere with her education.

At the time we had a large marquee-type structure that was acting as a temporary gym while our new chamber of torture was being constructed. The marquee had huge plastic walls that were tethered to long metal poles right the way around the sides. One night we locked the poor girl in, and in her desperation to find a light switch or a door she managed to dislodge one of the huge plastic sides which came swinging down and caught her a glancing blow on the side of the face, opening up a gash that required half a dozen stitches.

In fairness, you can't really get a more hands-on experience of treating injuries in the role than that.

She got a glowing reference from the club and left us knowing that her work experience (which was in tents – sorry!) had taught her a lot about the inner workings of the game.

How many fingers am I holding up?

The easiest targets are the best, and the easiest physios to wind up are the ones who take their job most seriously. They are the ones who exclusively deal in high drama, where every stretched tendon is potentially life-threatening and a tweaked hamstring could make a widow of some poor young woman.

To be fair, they are gripped by a fear that they might mess up and their mistake could be the one that will cost a player his career, and the physio his job. As a result they are compassionately overbearing and tyrannically caring. And we torture them.

During my career, back in the Dark Ages before concussion became something that necessitated being substituted as a mandatory precaution, I seemed to suffer more than my fair share of head traumas. Despite my ballerina-like agility I was always clashing heads and sticking my handsome face into places where I probably shouldn't have stuck it. More often than not I'd end up on the floor wondering who I was and not liking the answer when I figured it out. I never, ever suffered from double vision, only grogginess. For some reason I feel proud of that.

Anyway, this one particular physio we had would come screaming on to the pitch like a fire engine arriving at the scene of a blaze in a fireworks factory. Protocol alert! Stand back, everybody. He'd immediately hold up his fingers and ask me how many were there.

I'd always lie. If he held up three, I'd say six. If he held up five, I'd say ten. And every single time, without fail, over the course of maybe three years, he'd scream for the stretcher.

The stretcher would get there and I'd simply get up and laugh, walk off the pitch and wait for the referee to call me back on.

Football is about finding your pleasures where you can because sometimes, and especially in the heat of the battle, it can be all-consuming and too much to deal with. It was only a stupid little thing, but do you know something? It used to work for me.

Now that I think of it, perhaps I just thought I was lying about the number of fingers he was holding up . . .

This is going to hurt

The corner came in from the right and with one mighty punch our goalkeeper cleared the danger – and on the follow-through he broke my nose. After the game the physio took a look at me and, channelling the philosopher Albert Schweitzer (who famously believed you grew stronger by overcoming obstacles), said, 'Ah well, it builds character. Everybody should break their nose at least once.'

Call me pernickety, but this, to me, is the mark of a shit physio. My nose was pointing towards Manchester and the rest of my face, like my career, wasn't. I was fucked if it was going to stay like that.

A week later I was able to force the club to make an appointment with a specialist, and the physio came with me.

The specialist took one look and said, 'If you'd come to me the day after I could have reset this no problem. Or better yet, Mr Physio, if you'd gone on to the pitch at the time and applied some pressure to the joint then it would have clicked back into place. As it is . . . this is going to hurt. A lot.'

With that he asked me to lie down on the medical table in the centre of the room and without painkillers he put all of his weight on to one point of my nose and broke it in the opposite direction.

Today, when you drool over my matinee-idol good looks, you'd never know that it had ever been broken.

Unless, of course, you ask how I came through such a rough-and-tumble career unblemished, practically begging me to give you the album remix of this story.

I learned two things that day. Firstly, there are good physios and there are lazy physios. Secondly, nose specialists are infallible. They are always right.

They tell you that something is going to hurt and it fucking does. A lot.

OCTOBER

G host town. There is tumbleweed blowing through the training ground this week. It's quiet out there. Too quiet.

All the international players have been whisked away to the various corners of the globe and we are left behind with the long-term injured and a small group of young players and stragglers. It feels a little weird and slightly boring. We have enough to do but there's no urgency or excitement.

On the other hand, this is a good time for a little breather. Catch up with admin, spend more time with those long-term injured, do the odd bit of learning or a day course. The glamour never stops! In this room you are lucky if you've had a day off in the weeks since the season started.

Still. I'm bored.

The club's pulse beats to the regular rhythm of matches and the need to recover from one game and prepare for the next. That's what makes the place hum. That's why the club exists, the reason for us all being here. International weeks . . . they just seem to go on for ever! You are rested, recharged and

updated and there are still a few days before the full comple-
ment of players are back to amuse and annoy you again.

Perhaps it is unpatriotic and perhaps it's just because I'm getting old, but these weeks do nothing for me football-wise. My
main interest when scanning the match reports is checking
which of our players have come through unscathed and which
are now crocked. Naturally, if I read news of an injury I think
to myself that it would never have happened if I'd been there.

Not that I will get the complete picture from match reports
anyway. National set-ups don't like to advertise when a player
gets injured and is being sent back to his club with a problem.
Often the first we hear about it is when the player limps into the
medical room and says he won't be able to train today, he's got
a twinge here or a strain there. We don't like that much, but
managers hate it. That's why the player tells us instead of going
straight to the boss.

I do feel for the players. Only the lucky ones had a day at
home after our last league game before flying off to meet up
with their squads. Some of the South American players have
been playing in the Middle East, Singapore, Hong Kong and
China. That's a lot of time on airplanes and a lot of time zones.
The Asian players have a similar travel load. The Europeans get
off lightly in that regard. What makes it worse for them all is
that some of their colleagues who are left behind tend to get
quite a few days off. They jet off for some autumn sun and a
vitamin D top-up.

This is the second international break since the summer
tournaments, and that brings its own worries. Many countries
are starting their campaigns with new managers. National

managers like to show everybody why they have got the job so there will be brand-new training, and too much of it. There will be lots of shiny new ideas and systems to get used to. We generally have problems with national squad members when coaching staffs have attempted to justify their existence by spending long hours on the training field or doing intensive, exhausting sessions. During a season, our busiest periods for injuries come when players return from international duty. They are usually fatigue-induced ailments.

I just wish the national teams would be more logical and relaxed about their training.

A former Premier League manager once said to me, 'Players get fit in games. Training just gets in the way and should be minimal. Less is more. I much prefer two games per week. The week is easy: play, recover, play, recover.'

Simply put, the best policy for national managers is to pick players to play in the position and style they play in for their clubs. Find out what sort of training work they do at their clubs and then do very little of it during international week. Players don't like change. Players' bodies like it even less.

Many national managers, and I have to include England's recent ex Roy Hodgson here, work players for far too long on the training field. It's almost as if the need for recovery ceases when a player becomes an international. On top of that, the player is often asked to consider and learn new positions and instructions. The objective surely should be getting players on to the pitch feeling as sharp as they can and doing the things they are confident of doing.

These problems are compounded by national medical staff

who are all too willing to 'push' the players through the next game and don't give much thought to potential long-term risks. It's the club's medical team that has to pick up the pieces. Instead of communication and consultation we hear tales of players being encouraged to do work which tires or injures them. With some international set-ups there is a frustrating reluctance to get in touch with the player's club and have a discussion with the doctor or physio who treats that player week in week out about the best way to proceed.

There is another phenomenon that I associate with international breaks. Players carrying a niggle often find that the prospect of a few days off can speed up their recovery period.

The power of mind over injured matter!

Sometimes it's not so good being right.

A player comes a little sheepishly into our medical room, and we can tell there's a problem before he tells his story. He got injured late in the day during the first game of the two his country played during the break. He'd been moving backwards on his feet staying in front of his man, hoping not to buy a dummy. He bought a dummy. The opposition player feigned to go one way, but went the other. Our lad realized too late and tried to change direction but his right leg slipped and he fell over. The act of slipping while his body moved in the other direction led to him feeling a lateral force coming from the outside to the inside of his right knee. He walked off gingerly.

Back at HQ, we heard nothing about any injury.

What he has, it transpires, is a sprain of his medial collateral ligament, or MCL. Ever spent a few anxious days wondering what's stopping you from fully straightening your leg? It could be the MCL. It runs along the inside of your knee, and for those of you who were good in school, it connects the femur to the tibia. For the rest of you, it links your upper leg to your lower leg.

The match ended, and the team were thrown into a headlong rush to the airport for the flight taking them to their next game. Our boy got selected for a random drug test, and in the commotion, the knee never got the examination it really needed. Next thing he knew he was on a three-hour flight and wondering whether he should have said something.

His knee should have been immobilized at least with some kind of strapping or compression, iced and rested. He also needed to elevate the knee (in the usual way – not by taking it up to 35,000 feet). This is what we call the PRICE protocol: protection, rest, ice, compression and elevation. It brings down the swelling and pain around the injury, prevents further damage and minimizes the bleeding response.

Of course we have to factor in that players aren't the best diagnosticians when it comes to these matters. He may have declared himself to be fine and dandy. He had played well but had won fewer than half a dozen international caps so was perhaps guilty of wishful thinking. Keep quiet and it will all be OK!

Still, it's not too much work initially to test for an MCL sprain. Bend the knee and put pressure on the outside of it. You'll be able to tell if the inner knee is loose or painful, which would suggest an MCL injury. Hours later the medical team finally had a good look at the joint and tested how unstable things were. They decided to treat the injury on the road and not to put in a phone call to tell us what had happened. The club would have had him home on a private plane straight away.

Instead, he has returned to HQ this morning with his tale of woe. The manager has popped a gasket. Our sessions are meticulously organized in terms of numbers, tactics and specializations. People get very jumpy about last-minute changes.

We grade sprains on a scale from one to three. Grade one is the best news with grade three being the catastrophic end of things. It's not a precise science, but grade two might involve a little tearing of the ligament. Grade three can be anything from a big tear to a rupture. A rupture involves the possibility of surgery and may mean damage to other ligaments. What has happened in this case – and we have no video, although we are trying to track it down – is that the ligament has been moved too far and has been stretched beyond what it considers to be normal. Luckily it's a mild grade one sprain but we run an MRI anyway just to cover all bases.

His countrymen had dealt belatedly with the inflammation. It would have been preferable if that had happened immediately after the player came off. So now he is looking at a minimum of one week out, but it could be anything up to three.

Nobody is happy, and the next time he flies off to play for his country in four weeks' time he knows it will be like those times when he was a kid and wanted to go and hang out with friends his mother didn't approve of. He'll go with warnings ringing in his ear, numbers to call and a few things he needs to tell his national squad physio.

Sometimes the trust between a club or player and the

national set-up falls apart entirely. During a busy part of the season, players aren't too interested in travelling for international friendlies. They feel pressurized into doing something they see very little point in. Occasionally you will come under pressure yourself as a physio to provide a 'sick note' which might excuse the player from duty. Most top players carry around some form of niggle or ache which could do with a rest anyway so it isn't a big issue usually. It is quite easy for a player to exaggerate or even feign an illness or injury if he wants to, especially a flare-up of an ongoing chronic one.

Occasionally the country involved calls the player's bluff and gets him to travel to them so that they can check him out and assess for themselves how bad he is. This does nothing to improve relations.

The flip side is that sometimes a player may pressure you in the other direction because he desperately wants to go on an international trip but he is carrying a knock. That just means you must be more vigilant and specific when communicating with the national team's medics. This isn't always easy as they are elusive creatures.

It has only happened a few times, but sometimes the club will send one of us on an undercover mission to make sure one of our players is being looked after. The mission (should we choose to accept it) is to basically 'hide out' in the team hotel (or one nearby, but that involves sneaking in and out), see the player and consult and treat him on the quiet. Players often feel much more comfortable working with a physio they trust and deal with on a daily basis than submitting to a new regime with different ideas.

I understand fully why players retire from international football in order to prolong their careers. It's a long stretch, year after year mixing club fixtures with the need to be straight off to international duty for three to four weeks in a season, and then having only a few days in the summer before going off to tournaments. I can see how the novelty wears off, why they call it a day to be with the family more. And there is no doubt in my mind that with the intensity of the modern game players need to manage their bodies better. Those few periods of rest might add two or three years to a career.

Once in a blue moon a player might call you in confidence while on international duty and tell you that he is worried about being pressured to play, or about the way his injury is being treated. That can put you in a difficult position: you work for the club but you have a primary duty to that player as a patient.

At other times a player has come back and announced that his national physio claimed that everything being done at the club is wrong. Mostly you just take that sort of thing on the chin. As long as the player is happy with your opinion and strategy and hasn't lost confidence in the club's medical team, all is well. More often the players go along with what the national medics say just to keep a happy ship then slag them off when they get back.

I want to go home. It's past teatime. It's bedtime for the kids. But the young lady keeps pointing at her abdomen and making a face which suggests that she is either in pain, pregnant and not happy about it, or just overweight and wearing a blouse she doesn't like.

All the players have gone home. I don't speak Spanish and none of the medical staff who do are still around. My visitor seems to speak Spanish and nothing else. Also, I'm a physio not a doctor, so unless she has a hernia or a strain I wouldn't be much use to her even if I could speak Spanish.

I suggest through a pantomime of hand gestures, nods and repeatedly saying the words 'Wait here' that she should indeed wait there. I wander out to the players' car park and find just what I was hoping for. A player's wife. Or partner. Or mistress. Or sister. Or agent. I'm not sure. She is sitting behind the wheel of a huge black vehicle that looks like it was designed for driving VIPs through battlefields without having to worry about spilling their drinks. It's not a runaround for the school and shops anyway.

I tap the window. I establish that I am speaking with the wife of one of the players. The family's childminder was feeling ill, so Señora packed her into the car, drove her to the training ground and pointed her towards the medical centre. Ta da! Or olé.

Thankfully, she has decent English. She agrees to come in and act as translator but looks a little surprised that we don't retain a string of translators in the medical room just in case we have surprise out-of-hours visits like this.

When you deal with players, especially rich young players, the medical room becomes something of an A & E department. With so many foreign players around we are effectively a GP surgery to the mums, the grannies, the kids, the childminders, the cooks, the cleaners. We have all and sundry coming in. After a day dealing with first-teamers, the long-term injured, loanees, the chairman's best mate and then updating all the data as necessary, you can often be held back in the evening when family members and domestic staff start wandering in.

Of course it's unthinkable to turn anybody away. Many of the foreign players live in a bubble between their house, the club and a few nice shops and restaurants. Our job is to keep them happy in that bubble. A player who is discomforted or upset is bad for the club. And the smallest thing can make some players jumpy. Something small enough that it can only be measured using the tools of nanoscience can make a player's agent cross. The Yaya Touré Birthday Cake Tragedy springs to mind – the only instance in footballing history of a player's representative threatening to pull his client from a club because no one wished him a happy birthday or got him an iced sponge with a few candles in it. (Je Suis Yaya.)

The club has a full-time player liaison officer whose job is literally to keep players and their families happy, sorting out cars and bills and staff and flights. I've been at clubs where wealthy players have got into trouble for not paying domestic bills. Not having bothered to learn the language and having no curiosity when it comes to opening anything other than texts and Instagram messages, the bills just piled up in a drawer.

Simplifying the day-to-day lives of players is a vocation for some people.

If a top club signs a Spanish-speaking player – say, City securing the services of Sergio Agüero in 2011 – they don't expect him to integrate into the real world around him. Sometimes it happens, but most players see themselves as being with a club for three or four years and then moving on. When he arrived in the UK, Agüero, his then wife Giannina and those close to the couple were given mobile phones and laptops loaded with apps and info about every conceivable Spanish/Argentine-oriented activity for miles around. From language classes to flamenco lessons to tapas bars to Falklands War memorials. Any other interests were considered too. How to get to the local golf clubs. Where to lease a private plane. The stuff you and I take for granted.

Sponsors usually throw in a car or two at least until the player gets settled and starts his own collection. The car will come with a Spanish-language satnav and all conceivable destinations will be pre-loaded.

Whatever is needed after all this will be looked after by the player liaison staff.

If a horse breeder has a twitchy thoroughbred who needs to be kept calm he will put a donkey or two in the field with him. The thoroughbred's donkey is a trick football clubs have learned to deploy. If a club pays a lot of money for an overseas player it is often a good idea to sign a cheaper, less gifted compatriot for him to share lifts with, maybe even accommodation. Or get one of the less talented pros in the club to fill this void.

Pretty soon you might have a colony of players from one country, and then the worry is that they have become too strong an influence in the dressing room. And you start all over again.

For the medical room, all this means it's essential to have staff who can converse in the right language. We must also familiarize ourselves with the practices of players from different places – South Americans think it is weird to be asked to do weights, for instance; the French like getting massaged more than would be considered normal; and so on – and get introduced to their various gurus.

The travel we do doesn't broaden our minds, but the range of players we deal with helps to do just that.

Oh, and the childminder? Just something she ate. Dodgy lobster tail probably.

Players often get harassed by people who want to sell them certain things. Flash cars. Jewellery. Property. Incredible investment opportunities. I get bothered by people who tell me that the medical department will be a joke shop unless I buy some of what they are selling. What they really mean is that being able to boast that they have some kit installed at our club will be a big boost to their sales.

'You have to have this, mate. Seriously you do. It's a miracle worker that you just have to plug in. The blind receive sight, the lame walk, the lepers are cleansed, the deaf hear, the dead are raised, and good news is preached to the poor.'

'What's it like for tendons?'

'It's *made* for tendons. Did I not mention tendons?'

They never have research to back this up. A lot of their claims are based on pseudoscience and shonky evidence. I always take a deep breath and remind myself that the human body's healing processes are very good. Any other intervention has to be pretty nifty to justify itself.

A lot of the work we do is just making sure that things don't go wrong and the healing is going as well as possible. The Hippocratic oath of 'to abstain from doing harm' comes to mind. The challenge to speed up this natural healing process is interesting but not vital.

We are constantly being sold all variety of ultrasound equipment. Ultrasound works on collagenous tissue so it should be good for a ligament or certain tendons. All ultrasound amounts to is a soundwave which causes cells to oscillate. It stimulates fibroblasts – cells in connective tissue which produce collagen (the fibrous protein that is the main structural component of that tissue) and other fibres like glycosaminoglycans and glycoproteins – to do their job. Whether this actually makes the healing process quicker is debatable. We've been using ultrasound for about seventy years. There is still no hard evidence that it speeds things up.

A character in a Beckett play, the one where nothing happens twice (like last Saturday's draw at Boro), once said, 'Well that helped to pass the time.'

His buddy replied, 'It would have passed anyway.'

It's the same with fibroblasts. They are stimulated by the machine but they would have been stimulated anyway. That's what they are there for.

As physios, we have to come up with a thing called clinical reasoning before we decide on a course of action. We deliver a programme with numerous different treatments all of which have a small benefit, but when combined have a significant one. We weigh all the evidence, the research papers and your experience and decide that you need to take certain actions. There might be six different things you need to do for a particular injury in order to mend it. Some of those things will have good scientific evidence behind them, some may only be useful, and some are recommended simply because the player believes it is good for him and it makes him happy.

Or the player may have feelings about what is *not* good for him. You do get players coming in from time to time, and you break down their injury for them and outline the treatment, and no matter how extensively you explain the benefits of a particular machine to them they look at it, shake their heads and tell you they think it's a load of rubbish and they're not going anywhere near it. You can lead a footballer to a jeroboam of Dom Perignon but you can't make him drink (though he might anyway).

Electrotherapy, ultrasound machines, magnetic fields and magnetrons, inferential electrical current therapy, cryo chambers, vibration mats. These aren't a few of my favourite things. Cream-coloured ponies and crisp apple strudels would often be just as useful for effective treatment.

There are things which have made our lives easier, of course. The Game Ready is a portable ice compression machine. You can have it icing a player's knee on the coach on the way home from a match. So easy compared to faffing around with plastic bags. And anything that makes my life easier is an advance for science.

In longer-term rehab you treat progress as a series of stepping stones. One genuinely useful innovation has been enabling players to walk, run or sprint in an AlterG, a piece of kit that boasts 'superior technology invented by NASA, enabled by AlterG'.

As it happens, this boast has a basis in fact. A guy called

Robert Whalen designed a version of the machine for NASA back in the early nineties by enclosing an athlete's lower body in a chamber with a treadmill in it. Astronauts in a space station need to keep their muscles and bones healthy in a zero-gravity environment. Whalen's idea was that they should be able to run in a more natural way. Lowering the air pressure in the chamber pushed the astronaut down, simulating gravity and allowing them to run normally, and at their normal body weight.

The invention never made it off the ground (little aerospace joke there), but years later AlterG took up the idea and turned it on its head. They didn't want to simulate gravity, they wanted to take it away. The AlterG takes the weight *off* players recovering from leg and foot injuries.

It's a novel-looking machine – half treadmill, half bouncy castle. The player gets into a pair of tight neoprene shorts which have a sort of skirt attached. The skirt has zipper teeth. The player steps on to the treadmill, through a hole in its plastic casing, and zips himself in so that from the waist down he is now basically encased in an airtight plastic bag.

So far it's like a good night out in a Berlin nightclub.

The treadmill measures his weight, and the player chooses a setting for the intensity of the workout. I think these settings run from 'Neil Ruddock' right up to 'N'Golo Kanté'. The machine uses 'unweighting technology' to make the player feel up to 90 per cent lighter. Basically it inflates the plastic bag around the lower body and lifts the player off the surface of the treadmill.

The AlterG machine is used by a wide range of medical institutions for rehabbing accident victims, injured soldiers, old people and the overweight. It also helps neurologically dam-aged patients to relearn balance and gait after a brain injury. And most importantly for the future of humanity, it gets foot-ballers back on to the pitch quickly.

You can't move in different directions in an AlterG, which is limiting, but you can get the running mechanism right again without fear of putting your full weight down. Rehab machines go to 19km/h; others can go to 30km/h so you can actually sprint. If somebody has come off crutches they can walk at a level where they don't have to limp, and this helps the brain understand or recall how to walk without problems. Then, later, it's a great tool to progress body load in preparation to having a player run outside, again minimizing any limping.

Good buy.

We have NASA to thank for the AlterG, and we have the inventor of the atomic clock (Dr Atomic, I think) to thank for another key piece of kit. The GPS network is basically a collec-tion of clocks floating around in satellites. They serve up time and location information to us free of charge twenty-four hours a day, every day. GPS's ability to locate and track position has significant applications for sport. For some time we have been tracking players' movements during matches and training ses-sions. Coaches get instant feedback on distances covered and speeds attained. We know now, for instance, that even if Mesut Özil looks lazy he runs further than almost anybody on the field, game after game. Cesc Fàbregas at Chelsea does a huge amount of running too. Who would have known?

That is the most basic level of data, however. We are now using GPS to detect fatigue, building match-specific algorithms and assessing the activity loads involved in different positions. We are gaining real-time information on the physical capacity of our players and their contributions in game-specific training tasks, analysing what weight of hits they take.

In the medical room, though, the great benefit has been the emergence of running symmetry analysis. This new software identifies, quantifies and compares the forces at ground contact ('foot strike') on the right and left sides during running.

If somebody has an arthritic knee or an injury, they may not feel pain but nonetheless their body is offloading it. It's normal to offload a little, but you have to watch it. If you are doing a particular drill turning to the left, you may offload on to that side all the time of course. Now the percentage difference between the left and right stride is reported to the user as 'Imbalance'. A score of 'Zero' represents a symmetrical running stride where the weight on the left side is the same as on the right. A '5% Right' score reflects an asymmetrical stride, with a 5 per cent greater load on the right side compared with the left.

This is complex stuff. I have used it a lot on goalkeepers. For goalies it is important when jumping that they land with confidence. They may feel confident but I need to know that the distribution of weight is right. For an outfield player, deceleration may be the trouble. Slowing down very quickly is the biggest test for a knee. If you stop dead on the knee you are strong and confident with it. We look at decelerations over and over again until players can do it properly without a problem.

Specific tests for specific injuries for specific players.

Ah, when physios rule the world . . .

TSF: Second Opinion

My friend, the physio

It pays to befriend the physio. The physio is the one person you are certain to be seeing at some point in the season, when you'll have your cap in your hand. Depending on the injury you have picked up, he has the ability to make your life that much easier or that much worse. Some players are so brimful of their own celebrity that they are sniffy around all club staff. It's a short-sighted attitude. If you can fake sincerity with the physio you are always genuinely better off. If you actually like the guy, it's all gravy.

If you are going to be a dick, be a dick to the kitman, or the chef, or the reserve-team coach or the groundsman. The physio is your friend and your ally throughout.

When you are injured and lying on your bed of pain, the manager will generally defer to the physio when it comes to the nitty-gritty of what is wrong with you and how long it will continue to be wrong with you. All you have to do is lie there and look sad and enjoy the manager having one of those conversations where he is out of his depth after the first three-syllable word.

Befriending a physio also means you might be able to sub-liminally plant the idea in his head that it would be quite the medical innovation for him to recommend four days on the beach in Dubai instead of running and rehab in this hellhole.

The manager will duly oblige by taking whatever the physio recommends for the injured player at face value. The manager doesn't have the knowledge to argue, and even if he does, he doesn't have the balls to overrule the physio. Suppose the heap of expensive footballer flesh breaks down in rehab the next day when he might have been recuperating with maid service and mojitos?

It may feel like you are taking the piss, but seriously, you have to get past that. Nothing worse in the medical room than the smell of burning martyr.

If you come back all tanned and chirpy in a few days' time it gives everybody a lift, surely? You are doing the club a favour, and the physio is grateful to you for having freed up the time for him to do his paperwork. Good paperwork is at the heart of every great club.

You have had some respite, physical and mental, from the hell of it all and you are genuinely a better, healthier person for it. You say to the physio that you thought he was bloody mad when he suggested that you fly off for a few days, but you know what, mate, it might actually have worked!

Maybe it's just the delights of Placebo Al Mar, but on those occasions when I have been extradited to the sun I have always come back feeling a bit more chipper. Certain injuries can in fact be prolonged by living in Blighty, running around under its brooding sky and then lifting weights in a cold, empty gym.

Pins and needles

Occasionally you will find a physio fundamentalist who believes that every injury can be cured with one treatment.

It is usually acupuncture. I swear that there are physios up and down the country who believe that acupuncture is the answer to the world's problems, be they physical, emotional, financial, environmental or Kanye West. Acupuncture solves all.

I once saw three players each lying in state on his own treatment table and each looking like a pin cushion designed by Damien Hirst. Needles sticking like thickets of reeds out of their limbs. They had more holes in them than Arsène Wenger's argument for a new contract. As the physio was twisting the last one into the last player he realized that he didn't have enough to cover the area. So what did he do? He went back to the first player in the row, retrieved one of the needles, then walked back and finished the job. Even a heroin addict might have thought twice about grabbing a needle out of somebody else's thigh, but nobody batted an eyelid. Not the players or the physio.

It reminded me of a time years ago when the first influx of African players arrived at our club and the local private hospital, which we used for scans and surgery, developed a missionary zeal to bring enlightenment to these men.

A representative was sent out to give us all a cringey talk about the dangers of open cuts and the importance of not swapping shirts with blood on them, and how you should stick to your own towel when showering after training. They persuaded the kitman to sew our squad numbers into the towels in case we should inadvertently contaminate each other with the wrong skin colour. Your neighbour might end up with your yuppie flu and you with his malaria.

The gentleman giving the talk finished by stressing the fucking obvious. 'I surely don't need to tell you about the dangers of sharing needles. You are all athletes so I'm sure you don't go in for any of that. No?'

You wouldn't think so, would you?

Drugs and alcohol

Once upon a time I had a very nasty knee ligament injury. Cue violins.

The physio would happily drive me to the other end of the country to have prolotherapy, a fun procedure whereby you get an injection of sugary syrup deep into your leg then hope that the syrup reacts with the ligament and strengthens it by laying down new tissue and encouraging damaged fibres to knit back together again.

It was extraordinarily painful, but the physio didn't tell me that until it became obvious. His solution was novel. He found a pub opposite the Bupa hospital where the injections took place. The pub sold a choice ale by the name of Old Tom. Advertising itself shamelessly as a strong ale, what Old Tom hit you with was an eye-watering 8.5% ABV.

Two pints courageously downed one after the other took the edge off the pain caused by what the physio had blithely described as 'jabs'. They were actually violent penetrations with what felt like a javelin, not fucking 'jabs'. Frankly, four pints of Old Tom would have been better than two and would have served as an effective general anaesthetic for me. The physio claimed, however, that he needed me to remain awake so that the doctor could flex my knee joint against its natural resistance when we returned to the hospital.

I have very low moral standards and no self-respect and would have gladly let the doctor flex my knee while I was unconscious – but the physio was having none of it. Me being awake but plastered was apparently the best way of telling whether or not the treatment was working.

I'd feel better about myself if I could tell you that this was a one-off event but it was a series of injections and it became like a weird date night for me and the physio. I'd drink the drinks and then hobble straight over the road and into the doctor's room where he'd administer the injections.

That sound that was like nails down a blackboard? That was the needle on the back of my kneecap.

After about three months of drinking Old Tom we decided that this was not good in the long term for anything other than the development of alcoholism. Instead we were encouraged by the hospital to use Rohypnol.

Forget Old Tom, Rohypnol is properly scary stuff. But I did love that physio and still respected him the next morning.

What a stitch-up

In a Championship match I took a crack to the side of the head from a rogue elbow. We were a shambles in the game, absolutely shocking, and were beaten without offering resistance. That was our speciality at the time. The white flag.

After the game the changing room was like a graveyard. The only sound was the physio making enquiries about the exact source of the geyser of blood shooting from my head.

The manager stepped up to fill the silence. A volcanic man at the best of times, he was just about hanging on to his cool, but as the seconds ticked by he became unable to help himself. He warned us of his own imminent eruption.

'I'm going to say a few things,' he vowed, 'and it's going to hurt one or two of you, and you're just gonna have to take it I'm afraid.'

At that moment the physio whipped out the Vaseline to stem the flow of blood from my head. A fatal mistake.

'WILL YOU LEAVE HIS FUCKING HEAD ALONE!' screamed the manager.

To be fair to the physio, he volleyed it right back. This was some heroic shit. I say that the manager was volcanic. I actually mean psychotic but can't say that for legal reasons.

'WELL IT'S GONNA NEED FUCKING STITCHING, AIN'T IT?' the physio shouted.

It was like we were in a foxhole in 'Nam with Charlie pounding us.

Next there was an outbreak of fisticuffs. Eleven players stepping in. Well, ten actually. I sat there, a dishevelled kid and committed pacifist/chicken, waiting for the melee to die down.

(Note: Fights involving players or staff from any other club are generally dismissed as 'handbags' unless knives are drawn and throats are cut. Fights involving your own are deadly affairs and the word 'fisticuffs' doesn't really do justice to the violence involved.)

After about five minutes – which is a long time in fighting – there was a pool of blood forming around my feet, and I wondered how healthy it was to have more of your blood on the floor than in your veins. It wasn't the time to ask though.

The fight ended, everybody took their seats again and the physio retreated to the shower room, the safe haven of all physios on match days. The silence was eventually broken by the manager.

'TSF,' he said, 'you'd better get that stitched up before we get back on the coach.'

Fucking humanitarian.

NOVEMBER

This morning, late on in the training session, one of the reserves, a lad bursting to make a big impression, went over in a tackle. I saw the tumble out of the corner of my eye, but even if I had been staring directly, the view was obscured by other players.

I ran on. Usual interrogation.

'What happened?'

'I got done.'

'OK, but describe for me what happened.'

'He's done me. I have it and he's gone and he's done me.'

'OK, but describe what happened. It's this ankle? The right one?'

'Yeah, and the knee. Everything. I'm cattle-trucked, mate. Shit.'

'That bad? Do you have a next of kin I should call?'

'Fuck off, mate.'

'Right, well, let's get you off.'

'No, I'm fine.'

Two minutes later he was back in the thick of it, the whole episode completely forgotten.

I am either that good at my job or some players are complete drama queens. It is always essential not to panic and take your time when examining a sudden injury. You get so many false positives, especially with the lightweights. You have to learn to recognize the foolhardy heroes who would play on with a bloodied stump where their leg used to be and the poor snowflakes who think that every bruise is a career-ending disaster.

Players simply aren't reliable, even when it comes to their own wellbeing. For example, you know those questions we ask to test cognition? What day of the week is it? Who is the Prime Minister? Those questions are often a complete waste of time with footballers.

What day of the week is it?

Well, I've had three sleeps since the last match. Or is it two?

What is the Queen's name?

Beyoncé?

Who is the Prime Minister?

You know I'm Korean?

Oh yeah, so you are. What was the score in our last game?

Don't know. I didn't play.

For some reason we don't tend to video our training sessions very often. So if a player has had a knock in training it tends to be missed from a footage point of view. Which is a pity because in games it can be quite useful for us as medics actually to be able to see the incident that led to the injury.

The basic protocol for injury treatment is an acronym called SALTAPS. You may now take notes.

See – See the injury, specifically the mechanism of the injury. The situation, in other words.

Ask – Ask the player what has happened.

Look – Look at the affected area.

Touch – Touch the injury, meaning gently palpate the injured area.

Active – Can the player actively move the affected area?

Passive – Can you move the affected area? What movements can't the athlete make?

Special tests – Sometimes this is listed as 'Strength'. Basically, it means assess whether or not the player can stand up and walk with his injury. If he says that he can't move the injured area it can mean either that the player is just very anxious about causing further damage or that the injury is actually quite severe.

Essentially, you are trying to decide whether the player is safe and able to continue to play. If he can, that's obviously a good sign and the damage, if any, is minor.

(Funnily enough, if you check the FIFA website the first S is said to stand for 'Stop'. As in stop play if a player goes down. We'll talk about this later when we put tunnel doctors into the witness box.)

The trouble with 'seeing' the injury is that on match days your view is often obscured by gesticulating managers, timid linesmen, subs warming up and other players. None of them seem to realize that their principal duty on match day is not to get in my way.

Asking the player what happened is problematic too, as I've just described. Players tend to be pretty flaky documenters of their own injuries. It's either 'nothing' or a 'fucking disaster'.

So it really does help if you can see the mechanism of the injury yourself. A player will often think that his ankle or his knee twisted one way but the video will show that it went the other way. You need to see the reality of it if you possibly can.

From matches, we actually have a large database of videos – horror films of players getting injured. Watching them with a bucket of popcorn on your lap adds to your general knowledge of how injuries occur and the way in which players describe these events. Even with something as simple as a pulled hamstring you need to know if it was a sprinting injury or an overstretch. That can have a significant impact on how you rehab them and when they will play again.

By the way, we have lots of acronyms when it comes to treatment protocols. There's the basic ABCDE – airway, breathing, circulation, dysfunction (head injury), expose/examine (further injury) – which sometimes comes as DR ABCDE with 'danger' and 'response' added. (You can see what we have done there.) And of course the classic PRICE: protection, rest, ice, compression, elevation.

There is another rule of thumb, however, that I find very useful.

When you run on to the pitch, ask a player about the injury and try to assess him through his responses to your questions, any element of sarcasm or any hint of the player being a cock will usually indicate that he is fine.

'How many fingers am I holding up?'

'Thirteen?'

'You're fine.'

We have other little tests. Some players are catastrophists/ hypochondriacs. With the best will in the world, they will be talking bollocks. If somebody has back pain you know he is talking rubbish if he cries out in agony when you push down on his head in a movement with no physiological connection to the back. Technically known as Waddell's signs.

We test them to see how genuine they are being. Sometimes they just want to give you some bang for your buck.

'Does that hurt?'

'No.'

'Does that hurt?'

'Oh Jesus, yeah.'

'Hmmm, that's odd. There's no anatomical communication between there and where you say you are hurting.'

'Really? So is that serious then?'

There are gym rats and there are medical room mice. The latter are the players who are in with us so much they know everything. They know what fibroblasts do for a living and where they went to school. (Those of you who were paying attention while reading the October section will know all about them too.)

Sometimes players will show off by asking me to test them on the muscles of the body. They are so used to looking at the diagram up on the wall that they have inadvertently learned something. They know all the muscle groups. They tell me they reckon they could do my job. To retain my professional pride, I often need to make up a group in my head and ask them to describe its purpose.

Where is your Hebridean muscle?

We like to ask all injured players the standard question, 'On a scale of one to ten, how bad is the pain?' It's not too scientific an enquiry and it gives us a good general idea about the player. Most people never experience level ten pain but they don't want to choose a number too low in case we burst out laughing.

There are exceptions to every rule though.

Recently we had a player come back from loan for an assessment. He was injured.

Well, how would you rate the pain on a scale of one to ten, mate?

Most players, when asked how much pain they experience while playing, would be able to pick a number. Two or three. They can generally play with that level of discomfort. If they get to five or six they are struggling. Above that they can't play.

Anyway, when this player was asked, he said first that he just couldn't play or train with the pain.

'OK. So, how many out of ten, mate?'

'Not much.'

'So, five?'

'No. About half.'

'Are you sure?'

'Yeah.'

'You mean two point five out of ten, yes?'

'Yes.'

'And at its worst, how bad is it?'

'Ooooooh. Sometimes it's a one.'

It's funny, but we now had to find a way of getting him to

zero. Doing rehab with him every session he would do fine. Afterwards I'd ask, 'How do you feel, pain-wise?'

'About two?'

'Still, mate? You sure? You look fine.'

'Yeah. It's still bad.'

'You feel the same as in the games? That you couldn't play with the pain?'

'Yes.'

He wore the expression of a man who expects to be told that he has weeks to live. We did no manual therapy or manipulation. He went from machine to machine to machine. We gradually increased his levels of activity. It was a long process. It took weeks for him to acknowledge that he had zero pain.

Then there are players who take a minor knock and the one-to-ten scale lets us down again.

'How many out of ten is this one?'

'Nine or ten.'

'But you just walked in here without a limp.'

'Look, it's fucking agony, mate.'

People's interpretation of pain is subjective. Some players have three or four out of ten pain but they are fed up of treatment and tell themselves they will just live with it. You ask one morning how the pain is and they declare themselves miraculously cured.

We try to educate them about the innate healing power of the human body, teach them that they are going to be all right, that if they are just patient not only will they recover, they'll have a better chance of not breaking down again. Generally we get them playing with some sort of ball as quickly as we can. Not full on. I might start a player just kicking about with a little size two football, then maybe a size three or little plastic balls. This allows them to get the mechanism right and gain confidence before kicking the size five football. Then sometimes we'll put them in with one of the underage squads to let them rebuild their physical confidence.

It can feel a bit like being a vet. An injured horse can't tell you what happened to it, or how it's recovering from a knock. Quite often neither can a player.

We need to talk about hamstrings, the most common muscle injury in football. We have had a hamstring-free season so far so this may jinx it all, but I'm sorry, I need to talk about hamstrings. My wife's face glazes over when I bring up the subject. People on the school run who like asking me about life in the Prem move away if I mention the sorrowful mysteries of the biceps femoris. They don't know what they are missing. The hamstring is fundamental to everything in football. It's the smoke alarm that beeps when players are doing something they should not be doing.

A few years ago somebody noticed quite a lot of beeping at Goodison Park. Everton were seemingly in the middle of a never-ending plague of hamstring pulls. By early 2015 the club had suffered twenty hamstring injuries to eleven different players in the season and a half since Roberto Martínez had become manager. Martínez, who acquired a degree in physiotherapy when he was a player with Real Zaragoza, was quite alarmed. Everton were clearly either having very bad luck or something was wrong. The physio department was revamped. The hamstring injury rate has slowed, but looking at the last year or so eight players have been noted on PhysioRoom.com as having been out with hamstring injuries, several of them re-injuries.

Of course management and the style of training has changed in that period too so we can never know for sure what the trouble was. A change in a training regime can bring the plague on very quickly, or bring a plague to an end. Jürgen Klopp's early months at Liverpool brought a rash of injuries as the players were asked to work harder and run faster.

What we do know, however, is that hamstring injuries have plagued professional football since its inception. There is still no magic cure. No fix-all remedy. It's not getting better either. The incidence of hamstring injuries in sports like football has been relatively unchanged for over thirty years. Maybe because as we learn more about how to prevent them, the game continues to get faster and more demanding.

And the humble old hamstring costs money. Teams spent an estimated £198 million on injured players in 2014-15. That represented a 19 per cent increase over the previous five seasons. With today's wages, more than ever you want your top players on the pitch, not in the physio room.

The hamstrings – so called because butchers would hang a slaughtered pig by these tendons, as if they were strings – are the three muscles at the back of the thigh. The biceps femoris is on the outside, with the semitendinosus and the semimembranosus on the inside. Injury to these muscles occurs in sports involving explosive sprinting, decelerating and jumping actions (athletics, football, rugby, etc.), which put particular stress on the hamstrings.

The biggest problem is that there are so many different factors that can have a potentially negative impact on these muscles, ranging from fatigue and dehydration to having one leg longer than the other. There are three factors that increase the risk of hamstring injury that scientists agree on:

- Firstly, age: the older you get, the higher the risk.
- Secondly, having suffered a hamstring injury in the past – in which case you are more likely to get another one.
- Thirdly, and interestingly, any weakness in the opposite muscle group – the quadriceps.

You are also more susceptible to injuring your hamstring when you are tired and working really hard. There is a greater incidence of hamstring pulls in matches in the last fifteen minutes of each half.

Mild or grade one injuries comprise minor damage to a few muscle fibres or fasciae (connecting tissue) and may hinder you only for a few days. Lots of players can continue to play with a grade one hamstring, experiencing only 'tightness' or 'stiffness'. Or they'll just rest for a few days and, after some sort of tissue therapy (massage) or light pool exercises, come back for the next game. Luis Suárez is renowned for playing on with injuries such as a minor pulled hamstring, but maybe not Daniel Sturridge. It often depends on your character and pain threshold. Really!

It is important in the first few days of injury to do very little to the muscle and avoid further damage. We like to keep the area moving, though, so we use the pool a lot. It's at this stage that the clot or early scar is forming, in order to lay a framework for the muscle to heal. Just as a scab would form after a cut.

The No HARM protocol should also be applied – no heat, no alcohol, no running (or activity), no massage. This helps decrease the bleeding and swelling. Once the full mobility (stretch) of the hamstring is attained, and contraction of the muscle is improved, the rehabilitation process can begin, with both a strengthening and function-based approach.

Exercises targeting the local damaged hamstrings – such as hamstring curls and leg presses, and, later on, dead lifts, lunges, squats and Nordic curls – are combined with gradual increases in football-like running drills on the field, starting at low speeds to build tolerance and confidence before progressing on to sharper cutting movements and faster acceleration and deceleration drills. It is important to make sure that the hamstring muscle is fully capable of higher levels of activity before returning to full participation.

And it is clear from studies that if you run at 80 per cent, you will only stimulate the hamstrings by 80 per cent. If you want to make sure it is working at 100 per cent, you need to run at 100 per cent.

Once you are fit, you need to stay vigilant and keep the muscle strong and stimulated, either with a few high-level exercises or the odd sprint. For the first year after injury, the hamstring is three times more likely to re-injure.

I look around the medical room and add up all the years of science and study we have between us, and gaze at all the gleaming machines humming away ready for our use. Yet we are as defenceless against the simple hamstring pull as we were thirty years ago.

If you have never had a hamstring problem you will be oblivious to the entire thing and wonder what the fuss is about, but for those who have felt that worrying twinge, you are not alone!

At the training ground, it's interesting to gawk at the players' car park if you are a petrolhead. (Read on, you'll see the connection.) It's less interesting these days than it used to be, I'm told, now that the Jeep is almost ubiquitous. If not the brand, then the style. Players mainly drive big four-wheel-drive jobs these days. Dinky little sports cars have gone a little bit out of fashion. It was the humble hamstring that put paid to the Lambos, the Ferraris and the Porsches which used to dash in and out at top speed.

The thing about the sporty little runarounds is that they are very small and they get old very quickly (the cars, not the players). If you have spent, ooh, two weeks' wages on the latest model and then not long afterwards somebody trumps you with something flashier and sexier, the only way of keeping face is to one-up them.

The drawback is what your motor is doing to your body. Players don't generally live on the bus route to the training ground. They settle in clusters somewhere far away and often spend at least an hour driving to training and driving home again. They are cramped in their little sports cars, and if they are wealthy enough (they are), the little car that is wrapped around them is quite new and it has a brand-new clutch that is reassuringly stiff (though most footballers are too lazy to change gear and have automatics). Manual transmissions are bad for the athlete's body and particularly hard on the hamstring or sore knee tendon, especially if you're stuck in traffic. Famously, the small but perfectly formed Aston Villa full-back Alan Wright once strained a knee by stretching to reach the accelerator in his new Ferrari.

As far as I know, Ryan Giggs was the first top player to see the light. In his early twenties he suffered a series of hamstring injuries in his left leg. Somebody put two and two together and followed him to the car park. Aha! He switched to something a little roomier with a clutch that had learned to relax. He drove this for many years and the hamstring problems went away. No doubt for a while he was the laughing stock of the dressing room for driving a car that was more than six months old. He was Giggsy, though, and he would go on to play Premier League football till he was 103 years old, so the pack eventually followed suit.

Are all players created equal? Theologists and football fans have been asking the same question for a long time. The answer, if anybody had bothered to ask me, is no. And in football we don't even pretend.

If a player is a starter you know that there's a little bit more pressure when he comes into the room for treatment. I'm sure the manager loves all his players equally, but the ones who play week in week out are the ones who keep him in a job. He worries about them a little more.

And so do the board. If Sergio Agüero is taking home a £240K-a-week wage packet, somebody will soon be doing the mathematics if he is out for six weeks. That has a knock-on effect. Players know.

When he comes into the physio room the player who has been starting regularly doesn't want to lose his place. He doesn't want to give somebody else a run of games because he may never recover his starting spot, and management don't want the disruption to the team. There is a sense of urgency about the injury. So, in the only place that matters, all players are *not* created equal.

Another simple example. Your club meets at the training ground, or sometimes at a service station, to leave for away matches. If a squad player is ten minutes late, the chances of the team bus leaving on time regardless is high. If one of the substitutes for the day is late, the bus might linger for a few minutes, and if he is expendable the manager may make an example of him. If one of your superstars is late, the manager, or liaison officer, may text him, telling him not to worry or panic. Perhaps we can pick you up on the way?

And then there are the circumstances that can alter all priorities. A few years ago, when the club I was working for was approaching the defining fixtures of the season, three out of our four feasible centre-halves were injured. It was a period when the manager was spending as much time in the physio room fretting and sweating as the players. High pressure for everybody. And the injuries involved should have taken more weeks to heal than there were weeks left in the season.

We basically had four weeks to get at least two of the three guys fit from injuries that normally needed a minimum of six weeks. We did what we had to do. We were on tenterhooks. We couldn't risk disaster by overdoing it but couldn't undercut things either or they wouldn't progress enough.

I take it for granted nowadays that every player I treat is worth a few million quid. He has to be. As a Premier League player that's the minimum – no bargain basement stuff. So here we had three of them, and whatever their transfer value might have been, it was inflated by the pressure to get them fit quickly. What they were worth to the club right then was more than they were worth to any bidder. Fans sometimes think that players don't care. Those fans need to see injured footballers faced with missing the big games that they live for.

We did it. We finished the season at just about full strength getting everything we could out of those guys. None of the other players we were treating at that time would have been under the illusion that they were equal. We gave them what was needed as professionally as possible but we weren't sweating over them in the same way.

In football, how equal you are is determined both on and off the field. When it comes to a player who is new to the club we tend to screen him in pre-season just as we screen everybody, new or old, at that time. With the new player, though, we are exploring his capacity, his limits, his susceptibility to old injuries – discovering things we usually don't get to uncover at a last-minute medical. We are storing the data and we're making mental notes. He's a seventy-minute player. There are some games he won't have the intensity for. Thirty games a season if he's lucky.

It is generally not the player's fault if we decide that he isn't as robust as a tank. It is just the body he was given at the factory. Look at Daniel Sturridge or Jack Wilshere. Those poor guys have suffered more injuries over the last few years than some club squads have.

Calf trouble was the most recent problem to beset Sturridge. Throw in a couple of hip injuries, plenty of hamstring trouble, an oedema on the knee, a thigh muscle strain, a sprained ankle, a torn ankle ligament, a groin strain, one malleolar (ankle bone) injury and, just for fun, a viral infection. He is twenty-seven. His body keeps betraying him. It can't be much fun being young, gifted and crocked.

It's been interesting to see how, sometimes over the past few years, Liverpool have been at pains to stress certain things when notifying us all of Sturridge's most recent injury. If he has a strained thigh, Liverpool might point out that this wasn't the same problem as last time, which might have been hamstring or calf. Reading between the lines, I think somebody is saying that one injury was cleared but perhaps the player was not conditioned to cope with the training thrown at him. Hence he gets injured again, pretty quickly. The physio work has been done on the thigh to the point where it shouldn't be re-injured but the workload of getting back to match fitness has broken the player's body down somewhere else.

It bears repetition: the biggest influence on injury prevention are the coaches not the medical team. They organize and plan the intensity, content, volume and duration of each training session.

We sometimes forget that as a species we were designed to wander. We evolved as nomads, not cheetahs. We are designed to run and move at low intensity for hours on end. We aren't actually built for explosiveness. So the loads we put on players in terms of intensity have to be very well managed. With a guy who is injury-prone you may be getting up towards 100 per cent intensity and monitoring the injury you have just been treating, then lo and behold something else goes pop.

It can be heartbreaking for a player. And the physio.

The secret knack in this world of inequality – and I've said this before as well, but it too can bear repetition – is knowing precisely what to do in the days between games in order to prepare the player's body optimally for the next match. It's part science, part instinct and part listening.

I have long argued that football writers would be better people if they used the word 'morphotype' a little more freely. A morphotype is any of a group of different types of individuals of the same species in a population. Put cruelly – sorry, crudely (bit of a morphotypo there) – in football a centre-half looks like a centre-half, etc.

Eden Hazard would never be a centre-half, nor would he ever play in goal. He looks like a winger. Their morphotype tends to be specific to what the player is capable of. Theo Walcott, when you see him run, is also a winger. He could never be a holding midfield player. He isn't strong and stable enough.

Wayne Rooney is a different type of player from Walcott – always will be. Walcott is different from Hazard who is different from Zlatan Ibrahimović. They are all different from N'Golo

Kanté. It's a point I made earlier: training must be specific to a player's position, fitness and age.

Because, as we started out by saying, players are not all equal.

The season is in full swing now.

From a start where we looked ordinary enough we have hit a rhythm where we don't quite look extraordinary but we know what we are doing. It's like when the Beatles played three or four times a night in Hamburg when they were younger. They weren't famous when they started out, but they became a tight band, ready for when their break came. That's us. We're performing, getting good reviews. We're not moving up or down the table but if somebody else fails over the course of a weekend we move closer to the big time. And like the Beatles, we haven't yet suffered any major injuries. In fact we have one of the best records in the league in this regard.

The manager is happy. We know, because he dropped by to tell us. Whatever you are all doing, he said, you are to keep doing it. He escaped before we had the chance to explain to him in fond scientific detail exactly what we all do. You don't get that opportunity.

So, what makes a medical department successful?

Well, thank you for asking.

Is success measured on whether the medical team gets players back into the fray safely, whether a team has few injuries, or just whether the team wins trophies and it doesn't matter what the medical team do?

Good questions. I don't know the answers.

For instance, I enjoy stats and data but I have enough training and scientific instinct to have a healthy mistrust of them too. There is usually a flesh-and-blood story behind the bare numbers.

Does it just come down, then, to the volume of injuries?

Not quite. It would be simplistic to say that the team with the most injuries has a poor medical staff and those that have the fewest have the best. If this was the case, Arsenal and Newcastle United, who have consistently had a lot of injuries in recent years, must have terrible medical teams. They don't. And teams like West Brom and Chelsea, who have very few injuries, must have the best.

I have cobwebbed old colleagues who haven't been on a course in twenty years. They are doing the same thing they did twenty years ago. I like to know the latest this and the latest that, but being honest, 90 per cent of injuries get better on their own. Pulled thigh. Sprained ankle. Let them settle down and then restart things at a low level. They get better. You don't normally need somebody to get you through the process. A lot of quite lazy people make their careers on that.

Not in the Premier League though.

In the case of physios, most top Premier League clubs will employ up to half a dozen to cater for the first-team squad: there will be people with different language and cultural skills and also different specialities. Beyond that, a medical department consists of numerous doctors, physiotherapists, masseurs, sports therapists, osteopaths, podiatrists, chiropodists, psychologists and dentists. Some working full-time, some used as consultants. There aren't really any medical departments at top clubs where people just sit around smoking and playing cards.

Premier League clubs are in the business of assembling medical teams who can deal not just with the throughput of 90 per cent of common injuries, but who can make a difference with the other 10 per cent. Those players who struggle with a really bad injury or those injuries which don't heal in a normal way are the ones that need help. They are the challenging ones. Unless you keep up to date with the science you won't be able to see the wood for the trees.

There are two trending topics at Manchester United this year. Zlatan Ibrahimović is, it seems, better than we all thought he would be. He made it in all those other leagues but surely he wouldn't cut it in the Premier League? Like asking a highly paid cruise ship singer to perform at La Scala, we said. Many people had thought that Zlatan was just an all-singing, all-scoring personification of a busy Twitter account. But he can play. He hits the notes. He is a serious operator. And he's thirty-five and still doing it. Maybe Mourinho knows something after all.

The other trending topic is the long goodbye to Wayne Rooney. No sooner had Rooney reached his peak at a comparatively young age than the gods who giveth the hype started taking it away again and asking, is he really as good as we have been telling you he is?

That shrinking of Rooney's reputation only intensified with Zlatan's arrival. How come the Swede is so good at thirty-five and Rooney, who is several years younger, is being written off either for scrap or for China? Is it the damp air in Manchester taking its toll?

There are a few interesting things at work when it comes to player longevity.

It's always fun to compare players, but really it's apples and oranges. You might as well compare their hairlines. A player's ability to cope with a long professional career gets determined to a certain extent when he is born. Yep, sometimes it's just in your genes. Why does somebody die at forty-five when another person with a worse lifestyle lives into their seventies, and somebody else ends up getting a telegram from the Queen? (Does she still do telegrams or is it Snapchats now?)

I imagine we are not too far away from a time when major professional sports clubs will have scouts lurking around maternity units looking for those new arrivals endowed with the best genes.

If you've got the genes and the talent and had the good luck to be spotted, and to survive the academy system, the next barrier to longevity is significant injury.

If a player should suffer a catastrophic injury, it can work in different ways for him. Some players get an injury and are out for a long period. Nine months or more. In physical terms they might come back as good as, if not better than, before. They have worked really hard and in terms of stretching out a career they have made the injury work in their favour. A long-term injury is almost like a sabbatical in those cases. Sometimes a player can be out for a couple of years but he will go on and play into his mid-thirties.

For other players the opposite is the case. After they come back from injury they never seem to get themselves completely right again. It is tough to watch. Look at the unfortunate Andy

Carroll, always returning to battle, showing the old promise, and then breaking down again. He recovers, then he picks up another knock. Vincent Kompany comes to mind also.

Over a long period of time with successive injuries, a player's conditioning deteriorates and they never again seem to become robust enough to cope with regular games. They work hard, they push and push, but that's just how their bodies are.

After that it depends on what job you do. The position a player plays in determines a lot. John Terry is playing Premier League football this season at thirty-six. He's on the bench partly because he started the campaign injured and partly because of the system Chelsea have switched to, but he could still play if Chelsea were playing another system. He keeps himself well but he plays in the least functionally demanding position – centre-half.

For your modern strikers or wing-backs, physically their game is a lot more demanding. They struggle to extend their expiry dates. For a Robin van Persie or a Wayne Rooney, losing a bit of pace or conditioning is really noticeable. You can tailor your style but sometimes injuries hobble you, and sometimes you are just at the wrong club for self-improvement. Manchester United is too impatient an institution to allow even a legend like Rooney to slow down and learn how to contribute in different ways.

Ibrahimović is different. First of all he is a beast of a man. You can't coach somebody to be six foot four. On top of that he knows how to use his body to win the ball and hold it up while everybody else catches up. At United he surprised staff by finishing at the top of just about every strength and conditioning exercise they threw at him. That is work that a player can't begin when he is staring down the barrel of one last short contract. The earlier you develop good habits the longer your career will be. I know that for the last few clubs he has been at, Zlatan has brought his own man, the Italian Dario Fort, with him. In terms of the 'know your player' credo, having a personal physio is the ultimate luxury. Fort has worked with Zlatan in Milan and Paris. He knows where the borders are when it comes to pushing and preparing his client. The top players do that. Ronaldo is another whose chiselled physique reflects years of a near obsessive gym regime.

With the money in football, more and more players are likely to take that course of having somebody personally supervise their lifestyle. Three extra years at the top is worth a lot of money.

But back to Wayne and Zlatan. The Swede recently published a futuristic-looking image of himself working out in an altitude mask. If you are thinking of giving an altitude mask to somebody you love this Christmas, what it does is it 'helps to condition the lungs, in addition to regulating your breathing, boosting physical stamina and improving the oxygen efficiency within your blood'. According to the *Daily Mail*. So it must be true.

Of course at around the same time as Ibrahimović issued his mask photo, some pictures surfaced of Rooney at a wedding. He was drinking beer in the early hours while on England duty after allegedly being told to go to bed. Gareth Southgate, facing his first mini-crisis, said that England players could not drink heavily and perform well. If they chose the former they were risking losing their places.

The harsh fact is that if you take the really high-level Olympic athletes, their training regimes make it almost impossible to drink. You just can't put those toxins in your body and come out the other end and expect to perform. The drinking culture in English football has declined but it hasn't vanished. Players who enjoy a few beers have realized that in order to perform at the highest level they need to curb alcohol as much as they can.

There are some benefits to the odd drop of alcohol. How often the odd drop is enjoyed is the test. Some people cope with it better than others.

When we go out for a team dinner now, I look down the table and there is a lot less alcohol being consumed than there would have been fifteen years ago. Back then you would have had players literally sitting in the gutter after a few hours. I remember on one mid-season trip going for a walk with the manager the morning after one of these dinners. We walked past this crumpled heap in a gutter. The manager shook his head at the sadness of it. I said, 'Gaffer, that's your centre-half that is.' He looked at me, rolled his eyes, gave him a poke with his foot and said, 'Well, he's still alive. That's all right.' We walked on and got a coffee.

In recent years I haven't seen a player in that sort of state. They can't do it, and if they do somebody is going to snap a picture of them on their phone and stick their mugs up on social media.

The game has become more intense and demanding, but what we know about conditioning and how the body works has moved on too. If players do the right things for long enough their careers can stretch. Unfortunately it is easier to convince a thirty-two-year-old of that than a player ten years younger.

In the Champions League we usually play big teams based in big cities and backed by big money. There is an atmosphere in some of the great stadiums of Europe that reminds you of the luminous history of the team you are playing as well as the epic history of the competition.

Other than that, though, most Champions League trips are the same old, same old. There is not much difference between the Hiltons in Madrid, Milan and Manchester. These journeys are work trips. They are planned to keep players in an environment that is as familiar and soothing as possible. No distractions. No drinking in the local culture.

This week, though, we are in the eastern European equivalent of Leicester. A town that seems to think that modernization ended with the Soviets. As we drive in from the airport it is dark already (we have lost a few hours crossing time zones) and all we see are grey apartment buildings separated by streets of dirty snow. It looks like a town where it never really gets bright in winter, just less dark. And it is very far away. So far away that we left a day earlier just to get here.

We usually travel to away European fixtures on the morning of the day before the game, leaving the training ground or stadium as early as eight a.m., depending on how far we must travel. This time we have had to leave two days before the game, and we met at 6.30 a.m . . . and that was after an away league game at the weekend. I thought that my wife looked unhappy about it until I saw the faces of the players as we gathered. They were grieving. Most of them didn't know there was such a thing as 6.30 a.m. They normally don't drag themselves out of bed until after nine for regular training days, which start at 10.30 a.m. I kept hearing snippets of mean-spirited debate among players about Europe just being too big. Having to travel this far felt to them like victimization.

All the more amusing, then, to see their faces now, having flown back in time and landed at an airport which may have looked pretty swish in 1963. 'It's a fucking shithole, mate' is the most favourable comment Trivago could hope to harvest.

I don't often feel sorry for footballers but a trip like this is tough on those players who know in their hearts that they are unlikely to play. They have to keep themselves tuned in and buoyed up just in case, but really it's just a lot of time spent travelling to a place they have never heard of and will never remember having visited.

It's important to be in good nick, though. When we get to the hotel we set up a medical facility in a room that looks like it might once have been the presidential suite. We get to work on the tired and stiff players, and the familiar banter makes it feel like home pretty quickly.

If we win here we ensure qualification to the knockout stages with just a home game left to play in the group. It should be a tap-in for us but the unfamiliarity of the place is making everybody a little jumpy.

Our advance scout found this standard Western-style chain hotel for us a long time ago, when the draw was made, and the players have billeted themselves in here, closing out the cold and shuffling up and down the corridors in stockinged feet with headphones on and iPads in their hands. They look so sleek and tended and muscular, they could be a different species to the locals.

The team trains for an hour at the stadium the afternoon before the game. Stuck outside the town in woodland, it is a nice but very small arena. We establish the whereabouts of the local hospital and touch base with the local medics – a must in case we need help. Touch wood, the number of times I have had to take a player to hospital while away in another country is so low I could count them on one hand. I remember one preseason in Scandinavia and a player came over direct from a family holiday, and he was really ill from food poisoning. He had to stay in hospital, and when the team went home I stayed on for a day because nobody else would.

We try to avoid operations in unfamiliar countries as much as possible – only really in emergencies. It's not rampant xenophobia, it's just that you cannot control the quality of the surgeon or type of surgery undertaken very easily.

In fact, doing my work overseas can be a nightmare. We underestimate how excellent our medical facilities are in the UK, and trying to communicate with stadium medics with no grasp of the English language can be very difficult. At the stadium for this Champions League game there are a couple of medical staff with decent English. Hopefully they will be easy to find if we need them.

On match day after breakfast, with the players sorted and resting, I and a couple of the staff decide to take a walk into town. We spot a nice cathedral with colourful onion-shaped domes and the place seems to pick up a bit of life the closer to the river we get.

It is a rule on these trips that if we go out we must wear the club tracksuit, so we haven't gone more than a couple of hundred yards when we notice a few kids following along behind us. We flatter ourselves into thinking that maybe they think we are players. Seeing us stepping gingerly around town has surely made them confident about tonight.

We pass through a nice square which we agree would probably look lovely on a summer's day. A little further on I glance back to see if the kids are still following us. They are, except now they seem to have grown a lot taller and a lot meaner-looking.

'Look behind us,' I say to the others.

Then there's a shout that sounds like the battle cry of the Golden Horde, and instinctively we take off.

We sprint about a hundred yards until we realize there's nothing following us but abuse and laughter. We spot a large imposing-looking shop which seems to be dispensing coffee to frozen locals and go straight in and sit down at a long table near the window. We feel safe inside and try to convince ourselves that we sprinted here just in case the last of the seats got snapped up before we arrived.

Our pursuers pass by on the street a few seconds later, laughing and giving us the finger. As it turns out they aren't particularly menacing, but we linger over our coffees anyway. And agree that the adventure should be our mildly embarrassing little secret.

Leaving about half an hour later, we meet a small party of our own fans, dyed-in-the-wools who would follow the team to Timbuktu and back.

'Aye lads. Saw you boys running down the street earlier. What was all that about? Was it kicking off or something?'

'No! Just a bit of fun.'

'Want to watch it on these pavements, boys.'

They go on their way chuckling. They know that we are three scaredy-cats in tracksuits.

The game settles down early. We get an early goal and the wind goes out of them. They fall back into defence and decide that holding that margin in a dour siege is more glorious than trying to wipe it out with foolhardy attacks.

The only sour note is a late tackle minutes before half-time which tears a gash in the right full-back's ankle. Nothing too disastrous though. We take him up the tunnel and ask an official in a Champions League hi-vis jacket to open up the nice clean medical room we saw the day before. He glances down at the bleeding ankle and nods gravely.

Soon it becomes apparent that we are about to be blue-lighted in an ambulance to the city hospital. Not the best use of an emergency vehicle. There's a two-minute debate before the official opens the door to the medical room and tells the ambulance to go away. All through that debate the player has kept up a constant moan: 'I'm not going to the fucking hospital. No way. Tell him. No hospital.' I genuinely think he feels that if he does go he'll be left behind to languish there.

In the end the poor man in the UEFA jacket stands looking on in shock as we put five stitches into the ankle and send our full-back out for the second half.

We take our 1-0 and beat a retreat. We steal back three hours flying home over the time zones. The team sleeps. I hardly hear a murmur.

It's four in the morning when we get back to our cars at the training ground. It's back here for a light warm-down session at noon.

Sometimes they earn their money.

TSF: Second Opinion

And now for something completely different

Footballers are typical lads. Shock horror. And without wishing to lower the tone, I will now proceed to lower the tone.

There are many types of injuries. Some serious. Some comical. As a rule of thumb the more games you miss with an injury the more serious it is. Footballers' working knowledge of injuries is based on this rule. A hamstring injury can range from a grade one, a minor disruption of the muscle that causes some discomfort and gets you no sympathy, through to a grade three, a full-on tear of the same muscle that feels as if somebody has shot you in the back of the leg with an AK-47 while you're running away from a crime scene. Slowly. People treat you as if you have died.

After muscle injuries come ligament injuries. A medial ligament injury could mean three months but a bad cruciate injury could be nine. The worst injury a player can have, apart from something horrible happening to his spine or brain, is a tendon injury. If you rupture that sucker you are looking at a lot of pain and a year on the sidelines, and if you are any good the club is going to have to find a replacement for that year and you are going to have to pretend to wish him all the best.

After you've had your shot of pain, of course, the next danger you face is yourself. Even though, as Samuel L. Jackson has said about footballers, the path of the righteous man is beset on all sides by the inequities of the selfish and the tyranny of evil men, it is in fact puppyish overenthusiasm in rehab that is the scourge of all crocked players.

In the race to recover before they are forgotten entirely (or before the bank notices that they aren't getting bonuses any more but spending as if they are), players often over-egg the pudding, causing strains as evident as a poorly chosen metaphor about eggs and puddings.

There are, however, some life-altering injuries that are hilarious. I roomed with a goalkeeper once. But that's not the full story. Confusing me with somebody more sensitive, he told me how he had once strayed from his line to punch a corner that had been floated invitingly in from the left. The next thing he remembered was waking up on a physio table in the changing room. Several players had recognized the corner as a delicious low-hanging fruit and had converged with enthusiasm. The carnage had left the keeper with a bang on the back of the head and a bout of concussion which in my experience is no more serious for a keeper than when they suffered the same injury having been dropped at birth.

No problem, said the medics, there'll be other matches. You'll be back out there soon, smelling the smoke of battle as always.

A couple of days later he was in the canteen when the chef pulled him over. 'Your favourite today, pal – chicken curry with garlic naan.' (This is the footballers' watered-down version by the way, but chefs like to pretend that (a) it's gourmet standard, and (b) they have cooked your favourite just for you. Currying favour or buttering my parsnips. I'm on to them.)

The goalkeeper picked up the steaming dish of brown water and exotic spices plundered from Aldi.

Uh-oh. He couldn't smell anything.

The food footballers are served is so fat-free that you actually get more calories from the smell. But Chef had apparently forgotten to add any. The keeper asked him tactfully if he was using the right ingredients. The chef got the hump and said that of course he fucking was.

The goalkeeper invited the lads to smell the curry. He'd need their evidence if he was to litigate. The lads could smell the curry.

Yes, the goalie had lost his sense of smell. He couldn't smell anything. Not even danger.

Ten years later, trapped in a room with me, he still couldn't smell anything.

He explained how depressing it was to live in a world without scents. He was scentless. Food was less inviting. So was his wife. To his nostrils, a fine day spent rambling through Highland heather felt the same as a late-night chippy on a soggy evening in Middlesbrough.

I roomed with the poor man for a year, and it was only after a few months of our time together that I fully realized the extent of his loss. The simple but spiritually uplifting act of

166

catching my own farts in my hand and throwing them in his direction was entirely wasted on him.

I liked him but vowed to get a different room-mate the following season.

The pre-match fitness test

The pre-match fitness test is a comical piece of choreography.

Basically, if you need to have a pre-match fitness test then you are not fully fit. All parties know that. Still, the very fact that you are having such a test tells the world that you are either desperate to play and will die trying, or that the manager is desperate for you to play and will let you die trying. Not because he loves you. He just doesn't fancy the alternative.

Do you know how demoralizing it is for a fringe player to be told that he will be starting unless the first-choice geezer can limp fast enough come Saturday?

I have only ever taken part in three pre-match fitness tests. On each occasion I knew that I was almost indispensable to the manager, and he didn't care what sort of message he was sending to my keen young understudy.

The first time I had one was late in my career, and it was the most ridiculous of injuries. I'd slept awkwardly on my neck a couple of nights earlier and as a result I honestly couldn't turn my head to the right. This restricted me on the field and caused offence when the eyes-right command was barked while passing the viewing stand in military parades.

I'd had massages and acupuncture (the cure-all for everything in football), hot baths, saunas and steam room sessions.

Even a chiropractor had given me his best shot. The result was that I could turn my head about five degrees more than when I'd woken up two nights earlier.

The fitness test consisted of me heading balls thrown into the air by a coach. We deduced that so long as I didn't have to turn my head past five degrees to the right, I'd be fine. I could have fucking told them that before they devised the test and submitted it for peer review in medical journals. I played. We lost. I scored. We still lost.

The second test was many years later when I was north of thirty. I had damaged my hamstring. The entire opposition management team came out to watch this particular show.

They saw that I wasn't right. Even by their standards. I wanted to play but I was knackered. Every time I went to push off, my hamstring screamed at me to stop.

The following week we went through the same rigmarole but this time I was just about OK. I played. We won. I set up both goals. That was a good day.

I wish I'd made a little video of the test to post on Instagram for my audience of the previous week. I am a big man, but in many ways I am also a very small man.

If medicals are the black holes of football, then pre-match fitness tests are the ugly estates just beyond the black holes.

There really should be a cleverer ending to this anecdote. There isn't. I should have fitness-tested it before giving it a run-out. Apologies.

Bedknobs not broomsticks

What they don't tell you in *Gray's Anatomy*. That's right, the oldest one in the book isn't actually in the book.

Physios have medical beds with a hole in one end for the patient to push his face into as the physio cracks the clicks in the patient's back or soothes his hamstrings with a passive-aggressive massage.

The hole in the bed is an old idea that just keeps getting better as the world changes. I found that it was a good way to be on my phone texting my exotic but demanding Parisienne mistress while in the physio room. That would usually be a fine, but because you are face down with your boat race in a hole nobody sees you doing it. If you're not caught it never happened.

I had previously tried to lay a newspaper flat on the floor and peer through the hole to read it but my arms weren't long enough to turn the pages, and I figured that by the time I had evolved that capability the news would have grown stale. I'm no fool.

You need something to lose yourself in as the physio – or preferably the female masseuse – eases your tensions. The phone did that. App after app. Bad news story after bad news story. Angry incomprehensible text in French after angry incomprehensible text in pidgin English.

It all helped me to feel more relaxed about the situation. Until the big knobs took an interest.

The big knobs would wait for that little window of opportunity which opened when you weren't exactly sleeping but drifting somewhere in the fuzzy zone between reality and daydream. The biggest of the knobs would come to rest on your back.

That's right. I am literally speaking about players with big knobs here.

Sometimes they'd rub the python on the side of your face.

And if you were really relaxed they'd start smacking the thing against your forehead.

This is the shit that The Secret Physio won't tell you, but I bet it's happened at every club he's ever worked at. The trick is for the offender to keep going as long as he can before the patient actually comes round and realizes exactly what is happening.

Football being football, a player can be fined for using his mobile in the physio room but not for waving his cock around. The only danger he faces is from the experienced player who can pretend to be daydreaming only suddenly to spring into action like a coiled cobra ready to bite. One of my best friends in the game, a man who was more proud of his huge chap than he was of any of his huge cars, got his foreskin split after a lightning-quick strike by one of our ageing centre-halves. Nobody had seen the defender move like that in years.

For the miscreant, no stitches, but no blowjobs for a month either.

It's a tough game, the football, and in no way homoerotic.

Injury horrors

The ironic and sad thing about medical people is that they actually lack a vital part of the human brain. It is normal when presented with a mess of blood and guts to feel the urge to contribute something to the scene. Something like vomit, before passing out.

That is why humans were designed to keep all the blood and guts inside their skin. It's fucking gross.

Medical people are drawn to carnage and grossness like kids are drawn to playgrounds.

Some of the injuries I've seen are genuinely horrific. If medical people were normal people they'd have kept walking and just left the poor bastards to die. Who would have blamed them? Nobody wants to feel queasy before the Saturday evening fry-up.

Want to hear something truly shocking? OK, have somebody make you a cup of tea while you sit down.

I was once on the bench for a Premier League game. There you go. I warned you it would be bad.

Anyway, while I was unjustly incarcerated on the bench a top player broke his leg right in front of me. It was so sad. I sensed immediately that it could have been me and that the manager had left me on the bench for my own protection because I was too important to the team and the city.

Anyway (again), the poor fella didn't just break his leg. When he looked down, he saw that the top half of his leg was only joined to the bottom half in a reluctant way. Like how Scotland is attached to England. It was all being held together by one of our midfielders, who thoughtfully kept the man's leg in place until the specialists arrived. (Maybe our midfielder is missing that part of his brain too.) I heard him say tenderly to the lower leg, 'Look, don't leave now. Give it a chance. Everything passes. Except me. I don't have an assist bonus in my contract.'

When it happened I was in the doldrums of depression.

171

Charlie's Angels could have torn across the pitch in a red Lamborghini, flipped the vertical door towards the sky and asked me bare-chested whether or not I fancied moving to California with them because they intended to start a naked women's volleyball team and they needed a male masseur . . . I would have just told them to get lost, despite all the letters I had written to them down the years asking them to consider the idea.

The point is that I was depressed, and then I heard the crack. It was horrific and loud. Unmistakeable. I looked out from the dugout. The star's upper leg was pointing at me and his lower leg was pointing somewhere towards the Falklands. (That's still a patriotic thing to do. Who won that?)

The crowd cheered the tackle enthusiastically. Then they clapped the damaged and distressed player off the pitch to absolve themselves of guilt. Now how do you feel?

At the time I played for a team that made a virtue out of kicking the shit out of their opponents. I was there and I had to play ball but I drew the line at breaking legs. What do you feel when a player breaks his leg in Dave Busst style? Well, if you're as depressed and fucked off with your life as I was back then, you feel nothing. My first thought was one of a cold-blooded wanker: 'That'll help the fucking cause long term – he's a good player!'

It's amazing how conditioned you become to your manager's world view. It took me a long while to remember that winning didn't really have to look like *Guernica*.

That snap though. So loud that it stood out in relief against the crowd, which was at the time baying for blood. Our man who had issued the tackle made his own way off the pitch in a flood of tears. The victim left on a stretcher and wasn't seen in the vicinity of a pitch again for many months.

At that moment I remembered my dad telling me that he was in the stand when Tottenham's inspirational captain Dave Mackay, possibly the toughest man ever to play football, broke his leg in six places. My father said that you could hear the cracks all the way down Tottenham High Road. Mackay lifted himself on to the stretcher and was carried sitting bolt upright – no oxygen, no covering of his face with his hands, no wave to the crowd, no theatre. Mackay later said of the injury that only his sock and his skin had kept the lower half of his leg in contact with the top half.

They don't make them like Dave any more.

DECEMBER

It's too early to judge but we've had a run of decent results these past few weeks and the new manager seems to be a hit with the players, the staff and the fans. Just as importantly, the media see him as a good addition to the Premier League cast and the board are apparently walking around with Cheshire Cat grins asking each other the eternal question about who is a clever boy.

You are.

No, you are!

Fans will love anybody who gets results. The manager has changed things for the players, certainly, but he leaves them to get on with what they do. He treats us all with respect, he communicates and the people he has brought in with him are friendly and curious.

So what? Does it really matter? Well, it does. Players spend a lot of time in the medical room. Fit or not. It's the most social environment of the training ground. Trust and good relations between the staff and the players in here are really important. So while our relationship with the players is professional, it is different from the relationship the manager has with them. He has power. He has to make decisions that can change players' careers. We are just here to help the player get on to the pitch in good shape.

An insecure manager can resent the easy atmosphere of the medical room. He gets paranoid about the gossip and the chat and thinks players are malingering just to spite him. He starts seeing the medical room as a sort of lounge for disaffected players, and that maybe the medical staff are abetting the players in this.

There was a time when a manager had it in for a player so much that when he was injured (or malingering in the manager's eyes) he would make him come in for nine a.m. and stay until six p.m. It got to a point where if I had treated him any more I would actually have made him worse, so he would use the time to teach me how to play poker. I became quite good actually, but fortunately no gambling habit rubbed off on me.

A manager's hostility will then start to generate its own problems. People roll their eyes behind his back. He shows a glimpse of weakness and players are like schoolkids sensing the vulnerability of a supply teacher.

At a big club you learn not to get attached to managers. They don't last long. Usually they disappear without saying their goodbyes. It's a little like being a foot soldier in the Mafia. One minute your boss is a made guy with snazzy suits and a flash car and is calling the shots. Next day he's been whacked and you don't ask any questions.

Big clubs tend to whack their managers during the off-season but they plan the hit well in advance and usually have somebody in mind to step right in. It's only in the case of a complete loss-of-faith meltdown – Mourinho's second turn at Chelsea, André Villas-Boas at Spurs and Mark Hughes at City spring to mind – that a manager will be dispatched mid-season. December is usually the killing season.

Smaller clubs are more flexible about hiring and firing. The three- or four-game boost you might get from the arrival of a new manager in the middle of the season might be the difference between relegation and survival for a fraught club with a jumpy chairman.

So the bosses come and they go, and they don't get too attached to us either. But we're fairly sure our man will survive the December culls. Though we're not buying him Christmas presents without getting receipts.

I read a good book over the summer – *The Secret Race* by Tyler Hamilton and Daniel Coyle. It was a complete, in-depth, honest account of what the likes of Hamilton, Lance Armstrong and his fellow elite cyclists were doing in order to compete at the highest level of professional cycling in the 1990s and early 2000s. Taking performance-enhancing and recovery-enhancing drugs like cortisone, testosterone, growth hormone and EPO (erythropoietin, which controls red blood cell production), and even having blood transfusions between the stages of races in order to enhance their bodies' capacity to utilize oxygen and perform better, had become the norm in pro cycling.

The amazing thing is that many of these practices were commonplace and carried out 'legally' as they went under the radar of the drug testers at the time. The cyclists simply saw it as normal practice in order to perform at the highest level.

People often ask me whether footballers dope – for example, illegally taking performance-enhancing drugs (PEDs) to boost their recovery between games and optimize their performance. In short, I have never seen a player take a PED or heard substantial rumours about it. It just doesn't happen in football in the UK.

I have heard of illegal practices at European clubs where players are given intravenous drips at half-time and intramuscular injections to speed up injury recovery. There were murmurings a couple of decades ago about Marseille players having been injected before the 1993 Champions League final against AC Milan, but they remain rumours.

Tyler Hamilton was a prosecution witness in the Operation Puerto doping case in Spain. Dr Eufemiano Fuentes, the medic at the centre of the case, claimed that he worked for players at several big clubs, but as of yet no players have been pursued.

When players arrive here in the UK from some European clubs, they are often surprised that our doctors will not administer medications that they have received previously. We have a good system here in the UK . . . but is it excessive?

In 2011-12, the FA carried out 1,278 drug tests. Only four of them were positive. Yes, it is extremely important to keep football clear of illegal drugs in order to protect the players and keep an even 'playing field', but most of these positive tests were for recreational drugs, like cocaine, or because a player had accidentally taken a medicine, such as a nasal spray, with a mild stimulant in it.

I repeat, I have never seen or heard of players taking amphet-amines, EPO or steroids in order to perform better.

Cocaine is banned in both professional and amateur sports, but given their lifestyle it would be surprising if some players weren't tempted to dabble. Chelsea sacked Adrian Mutu back in the early noughties after he tested positive for the drug. When testing is done regularly, it is easy to detect a cocaine user – the substance is readily traceable in the urine up to five days after use. Given the risks involved for a player I imagine that cocaine use would be restricted to the occasional off-season holiday.

Still, in football as in all sports, drug testing has become a fact of life for players. They always moan about it but they know it has to be done. Whenever a player thinks that testing is exces-sive and intrusive you need only ask what he would think if he heard rumours that a rival team were doping. Within seconds he'd be calling for more stringent doping controls. Many play-ers and athletes who see testing as a nuisance need instead to see it as something that protects not only them from cheats but their sport as a whole.

Tests aren't carried out that often, perhaps once every month or so at the training ground and at big games. Of course it is annoying when you win a marquee fixture, maybe a cup final, and a couple of your top-name players aren't in the changing room celebrating with their team-mates because they're in the doping control room desperately trying to pee. And the physio is stuck there too, drumming his fingers, waiting for the players to perform when he knows not only that he's missing all the dressing-room fun, but he's got work to do as well, and every-one will soon be desperate to get on the coach home.

Players can be tested by the FA or, if they are in Europe, by UEFA, and have to give blood as well as urine samples. Although it's random, some players do seem to get picked out more than others – and if that happens they can easily feel as though there's a conspiracy against them.

Tests can occur at any time and are usually carried out on training days. Random testing that takes place outside training will become more common, though. We will see more cases where the tester will just turn up unannounced at a player's home. They won't like that.

Players must give their whereabouts for a certain hour of the day if they are not present at training. Many players have no idea about this because the club's admin staff do it for them, but I have seen a few players who, at the last minute, go sick or are given personal leave – and they have not given an alternative time or place for where they will be. Players even have to tell the authorities if they are taken to a pool off-site for rehab, or they leave early – a similar scenario to the one that led to Rio Ferdinand's ban a few years ago. Or . . . was he hiding something? If you make a mistake the rumours will follow you around for a long time in the modern climate of mistrust.

When a player is pulled for testing, the club doctor or physio may accompany him to doping control. This is necessary as the player usually hasn't got a clue what he has been taking. The player forgets that it is *his* responsibility not only to inform the authorities of his whereabouts but to remember what medication he is taking as well. It is a common misconception (usually by naive players) that if the doctor says it's OK to take a medication, that's OK. It's not their fault if they get a positive test, it's the doctor's. Wrong. The doctor or physio can advise the player on what to take but, ultimately, the responsibility lies 100 per cent with the player.

Of course we are very careful about what we administer at the club, but many players listen to advice from other players and 'gurus' and may quite innocently be taking something which is on the banned list because it contains an illegal stimulant. Taking supplements can be risky. Some are made in factories where banned substances are also made and traces of those substances can get into the so-called 'safe' product. An analysis of 634 supplements by the IOC in 2002 found that 94 had banned substances in them without any indication on the label. Some even contained traces of glass, and one had faeces in it. I always ask a player if what he is taking is worth it. What's the benefit? Is there a safer, diet-controlled method of supplementing instead? Often there is.

Am I naive about the levels of drug use in our game? I don't think so. In football, the level to which performance enhancement is useful is limited. Skill and footballing intelligence can't be artificially enhanced. A player may run 12 to 14km in a game but that is over ninety minutes with a break in between. That is not elite Olympian pace or anywhere near it. An elite marathon runner clips along at over 20km/h non-stop for just over two hours. Of course what he or she isn't doing is all the turns, cuts, accelerations and decelerations a footballer is doing, alongside execution of ball skills. PEDs won't help with technical ability. The benefits in running, cycling or swimming are pretty clear, but if you are a footballer, EPO won't give you a Cruyff turn.

There are advantages to be had from using PEDs if you are a player, but the gains in terms of your cardiovascular performance are limited, and the consequences of getting caught are catastrophic for player and club. The occasional player might take the risk out of ignorance but nobody in a medical room would. We live and work cheek by jowl. We even room in pairs.

While there is not a problem with footballers taking performance-enhancing drugs – as far as I have seen – there is regular abuse of legal medications. This can be seen in the excessive use of anti-inflammatories such as Voltarol and ibuprofen, mild painkillers such as paracetamol and the handing out of antibiotics at the first hint of an infection.

I've seen many players taking these medications for training. Sometimes they've bought the drugs themselves; often they have been given to them by physios or doctors only too happy to get the player out on the field. The player is simply asked 'Do you want an anti-inflamm?' and the player accepts. No discussion of why, or what the problem is, or whether it's necessary; no exploration of the possibility that there's another way of treating the issue. Sometimes it even becomes a habit to take a tablet for training. Do they improve healing? Now, doctors are moving away from anti-flamms because they feel they hinder the healing process more than they help with pain control. So a paracetamol might be given instead of an ibuprofen.

The former Liverpool player Daniel Agger gave an interview to a Danish newspaper last year. Most English papers picked up on it of course. Agger's words should be pinned somewhere on every dressing-room wall.

He described a game in March 2015 when he was captain of Brøndby in the Danish league. Less than half an hour into the game he could play no more. He came off and collapsed in the physio room.

By then Agger had developed an anti-inflamm habit. For a long period of his career he'd taken a lot of anti-inflammatories, frequently exceeding the recommended dosage.

The events that brought the problem to a head will be familiar in some form to most players. A week before the game (against Copenhagen) Agger was suffering from a knock and was rated doubtful. He wanted to play, as every player does. For a week he took the maximum recommended dose of the anti-inflamm in the knowledge that it was dangerous to hit that limit for more than three days. On the day of the game, he had taken four pills by the time he arrived for the pre-match meeting. He fell asleep on the coach to the stadium and had to be shaken awake. In the dressing room he took a caffeine shot and an energy drink before heading out for the warm-up. He gave a rambling pep talk. When the game started he felt wretched. He attempted a header early on but missed the ball, which hit him on the arm. Not long after that his body gave up.

In his long and often heroic Anfield career, Agger had become accustomed to pain. His fundamental physical problem is that he is hypermobile – that is, his joints overextend. He developed back trouble after a fall on a pre-season trip to Asia in 2008. He eventually suffered a prolapsed disc in his back, prompting pain in his knees and toes. He reckons that in his final two years with Liverpool he was performing to only 70 or 80 per cent of his ability.

When he returned to Denmark his condition got worse. In order to play he took anti-inflammatory drugs, often Celebrex, which is used to treat rheumatism. He was, as we've seen, cavalier about exceeding the recommended maximum dose.

Agger stopped taking anti-inflammatories after the Brøndby incident, but he knew the damage was done.

Will there be numerous former players in ten to twenty years' time complaining of liver and kidney problems thanks to excessive use of anti-inflamms? Doctors are widespread in the game now and of course we are the better for their specialist knowledge. But when I began in football a club might have had a relationship with a local GP and that was about it. So many doctors working for clubs has meant a flood of easy-to-access prescriptions. At one club I was at a player used to help himself to the medicine cabinet, not always with the doc's knowledge. This may have led to a serious illness he later had.

Research is revealing the patchy record of anti-inflammatories and corticosteroid injections. Corticosteroids, which basically stop inflammation in its tracks so that there is no chance for the process to continue, are used a lot more sparingly these days. They can be used for chronic issues where getting rid of the local inflammation removes the pain, but only if you also address the cause. Twenty-five or thirty years ago, players knew that cortisone injections worked as pain relief and would have one before every match. Today, many of those players are applying for blue parking permits as their muscles are destroyed.

Evidence may now show that anti-inflamms could be detrimental to the healing process, but still players like Daniel Agger become dependent on them. Sometimes because they are creatures of habit and don't like changing what has worked in the past, sometimes because they think they are being brave professionals and presenting themselves to play when they really should not. Maybe in years to come players will be suing doctors for medical conditions linked with the long-term medications they took.

The way that footballers relate to staff has changed a bit during my time in football. I blame the money that has come into the game. Where you were once a friend you are now an employee. Which isn't always a bad thing: it's good to keep a professional distance. Lots of people come to work at football clubs because they are fans and they end up getting burned when they think they have established a social relationship with a player.

There are still quite a few of them who are decent blokes you can build a rapport with, even though they are multi-millionaires. Naturally, you occasionally get a big-time Charlie (or Carlos) who sees himself as a cut above everybody else. They look down on individuals, not just in the medical room but even in the dressing room. Good luck to them. What they miss out on is punishment in itself.

In the lower leagues it was different. There was more parity and a sense that we were all in it together. At the Premier League level the players are in a different financial stratosphere. There is disparity between the management, the players and staff. Gone are the days when a manager gets paid more than the players.

I'm not complaining about how much money players earn. If that money is coming into the game they are the ones who should earn it. But some of the players can be moody pricks. The captain, for instance, isn't a morning person. No point in talking to him before lunch. Then when he wants to talk to you he can be fine. You feel like an employee in the morning, a mate in the afternoon.

You have to appreciate too that it's not always personal. There are some players for whom the last place in the world they want to be is the physio room. They express that through the medium of treating you like shit.

Phones have changed relationships within the club too. They aren't banned (I have seen situations where they are banned and it is hard to enforce). Still, does a player have to be welded to the thing at all times?

Many players no longer live in the moment, they are just tweeting and texting constantly. They walk out into stadiums and they're taking selfies. Their match is going to be on television, they are surrounded by professional photographers, and they have to have selfies to tweet or send to friends as if they need to prove that they have been there.

It's the same in the physio room. You walk in and there might be six players on beds getting treatment and each one of them will be engrossed in his phone while being attended to. They're not talking to each other, they're not talking to the staff. Their minds aren't even present.

Before games too they are entranced by their phones. I find it incredible. You can walk into a dressing room these days and every player will be hunched over his device, and will probably have headphones on as well just to isolate himself further. Then a few minutes later they get in a huddle and promise to go out and die for each other.

The modern footballer is lithe and muscular, graceful and sleek, coiled like a spring and trained to react a split second before most people even realize what is happening. I'd like to take this opportunity to recount some of their superpowers here . . .

Let's start with goalies, the most feline of footballing athletes. The Spanish keeper Santiago Cañizares missed the 2002 World Cup finals. He dropped a bottle of aftershave into a sink in his hotel room. It shattered, and a piece of glass fell on one of his feet, severing a tendon in a big toe. Dave Beasant, once of Wimbledon and Chelsea, did a similar thing, though with the aid of a bottle of salad cream. His severed big-toe tendon ruled him out for eight weeks.

Years ago, Brentford goalie Chic Brodie ended his career when he collided with a dog that had run on to the pitch. The dog got the ball. Chic shattered his kneecap. He noted that 'the dog might have been a small one but it just happened to be a solid one'. The dog signed a three-year contract with the club the following week.

David James, the England goalkeeper, once pulled a back muscle when reaching for the television remote control. James was also a keen angler and on one occasion tweaked a shoulder when trying to land a massive carp. Or maybe it was just small but solid.

Alex Stepney, Manchester United's keeper in the seventies, dislocated his jaw while shouting at his defenders during a match against Birmingham City. American goalie Kasey Keller knocked out his front teeth while pulling his golf clubs out of the boot of his car. Michael Stensgaard, the Danish goalkeeper, was forced to retire after suffering a shoulder injury as he daringly attempted to fold down an ironing board.

Footballers should opt for the full hazmat when dealing with babies. Kevin Kyle, the Kilmarnock striker, spent a night in hospital in 2006 when his eight-month-old son kicked a jug of boiling water over his crotch, lightly broiling the meat and veg. Mansfield's Adam Chapman once shook a hot bottle of milk he had just prepared for his infant. He'd forgotten to screw the lid on and ended up with a scalded nipple.

The world is a minefield that footballers have to negotiate daily. Ecuador's Enner Valencia once lacerated a big toe by standing on a broken teacup. Derek Lyle, the Dundee striker, fell through a glass table at his home. Or did he dive, ref? Either way he needed sixteen stitches in a stomach wound and missed a Scottish Cup quarter-final against Queen of the South.

Charlie George, the Arsenal legend of yore, cut off a toe with a lawnmower (one of his own toes). Lee Hodges, of Barnet, slipped on a bar of soap in the shower and wrenched his groin. When Rio Ferdinand was at Leeds United, he sat for too long in one position while watching TV and picked up a knee tendon strain.

Special mention to England midfielder Alan Mullery who missed a 1964 tour of South America having suffered a landmark injury: he damaged his back while brushing his teeth.

Aston Villa's Darius Vassell once pierced his toenail with a domestic power drill. He thought it might relieve the pressure on a swollen toe. When there is a build-up of blood under a nail it can be treated by drilling a small hole and releasing the pressure, but only in a sterile environment, and only if the drill is a specialized tool in the hands of a trained professional. Black & Decker had never thought to put a warning on packaging about the inadvisability of using their power tools to perform minor surgery on yourself. Darius wound up with an infection.

Most of these things happened before players even got on to the pitch and started bumping into each other. Once they do, it gets worse. Tony Adams dropped Steve Morrow on the grass while the pair were celebrating Arsenal's 1993 League Cup win. (I presume Adams had one arm up calling for offside, as was his wont.) Morrow landed awkwardly on his arm and broke it. Liverpool medics Andy Massey and Chris Morgan had to stitch up Steven Gerrard's penis after it suffered a laceration in a cup game against Bournemouth. Four stitches, in case you are wondering. The medic/player relationship has seldom had its foundation of trust so severely tested. Still, the incident brought forth a beautiful piece of prose in Gerrard's autobiography. 'My dick was stinging like fuck,' he recalled. It might be all worth it just to record in the medical notes that the patient presented with an ailment which was described thus.

Andy Carroll once injured a knee after catching his foot in a net while collecting balls during training. Andy is so injury-prone the knee was going to get busted anyway. It was just a surprise that it was a net that did the honours.

Then you have all the injuries that players pick up while playing golf too poorly or tennis too vigorously, having sex too poorly *and* too vigorously, or while indulging in countless other leisure pursuits.

Worrying about all these things has made me old before my time. It's such a relief when I see a player pull into the car park and negotiate his way to the dressing room safely.

Today's weather forecast says we are to expect snow. Please, no. They can't be expected to cope with slippery surfaces as well as all the other dangers.

Folks, let's be careful out there.

We played Sunderland the other night in the icy confines of the Stadium of Light. Then yesterday we had an Under-23 match against Reading. For the Under-23 game we had seven first-team players playing, five of them senior internationals. A reserve fixture is nothing like playing a real game, but afterwards some of them said that they felt a bit stiff. They hadn't done that for a good number of weeks. They have all been fit according to the charts and indexes we keep, but they haven't been playing matches. Why? The same eleven keeps being put out for as long as we keep this decent run going. Until somebody gets injured or struggles, that's how it will be.

A player's attitude to having the chance to feature in the odd reserve game varies of course. Some players won't touch them with a bargepole. We tend to give them the option because there's nothing worse than pushing a player out there if he really doesn't want to play. He'll drag everybody else down into his sulky mood. And of course the less committed he is to the idea the better chance he has of picking up an injury. You don't want to be reproached with that afterwards. But this week, as I said, seven good first-team players requested to play. Quite unheard of. The match was at the training ground on the academy pitch and they were all desperate for a game. It helped too that the manager was around. If it had been an away fixture at Hartlepool they might have felt a little differently.

Hark! I can hear carol singers at the door. I leave my chestnuts roasting on the fire and I go out to watch. Lo, it is a group of ruddy-faced Prem managers singing a yuletide favourite.

> O Fixture List!
> O Fixture List!
> We're all being killed,
> by the fixture list.

I grab my shotgun and tell them to get off my land. 'You haven't three wise men between you!' I shout. 'The bloody fixtures are the same for everybody. Just get on with it!'

The Christmas and New Year schedule is the most intensive period of the season with matches every few days. This year is no different. Why complain? It's football, but it's the entertainment industry in England. Holiday time for the muggles is the busy time for the game. They didn't change to a packed end-of-year schedule just to spite you personally.

But yes, it's tough, especially for those of us with families, as you are usually working during all the bank holidays, including Christmas Day, Boxing Day and the turn of the New Year. The fixtures can be a little harsh if you have an away game on 26 December. That means you train lightly and travel to an overnight hotel on Christmas Day, or Christmas night. You have to have a very understanding spouse . . . and kids!

With the games coming thick and fast, there is no time for intensive training. You are just patching players up for the next match in a few days. Many players won't train at all between games, especially if they have long-term problems that can't take two or three games in seven days as well as training.

Optimal recovery is essential. There are no concerns over not refuelling enough during the festive period, but keeping to the right foods and avoiding too much alcohol is paramount. Players from different countries do things differently, but the British lads tend to shoot off after training on Christmas Day as this is their day, or half day, with the family.

Working in football means no drinking on Christmas Day or Boxing Day. You open the presents with the kids before going to work on Christmas Day, or when you get home later. Maybe you do it before going to the hotel with the team on Christmas night. Fitting in some kind of dinner somewhere is the problem. It all comes with the territory though.

I make brief appearances at the family get-togethers if possible, sticking my head into a roomful of friends and relatives as I pop by each house and get ready to leave again. They understand. They don't complain. Maybe they don't actually like me that much.

By way of festivities at the club, there will usually be a Christmas dinner at the training ground for all the staff and unenthusiastic players at some point. This is a duty rather than a pleasure – just a glorified lunch really. Nobody gets tucked into the vino as we still have jobs to do afterwards. We tend to let our hair down a little more in the evenings arranged over Christmas especially for medical staff, with or without spouses.

Of course players usually have an evening Christmas do themselves. These used to be legendary occasions of debauchery and scandal, but they are not as popular as they used to be. Teams have become more multinational and many players don't drink at all so those shindigs have become a lot tamer.

Traditionally, the one match we all really hate is the one that sometimes gets squeezed in between Boxing Day and New Year, generally around 28 December. That's a killer, sandwiched between two holidays and with only forty-eight hours between fixtures. If I was a betting person I would place my money on a series of draws in the games around the 28th. Teams are tired and there is a feeling of truce in the air.

This year, though, New Year's Eve falls on a Saturday, which means most of us will work on Boxing Day, a Monday, and not again until Saturday. The downside is that most of us are playing again on the Monday of the following week. And at the end of that week it's FA Cup time.

It's a time of year, though, when you can expect fond seasons greetings from former club players who have moved abroad to play. They send Instagram pictures of themselves on holiday in Dubai or Bali with their families. Happy Winter Break, they say.

Then – oops, completely forgot you guys don't get a winter break!

TSF: Second Opinion

A little white lie

Do you remember the player who tripped over his dog at home? His ankle swelled up and the pain was so great that when the manager asked why he stank of booze at training, he replied that he'd had to drink some whisky to numb it. Remember?

What actually happened was that he fell down some steps outside a nightclub after drinking the place dry.

Remember now? So do I. Painfully.

Mad injuries

I've always been the adventurer. Half Indiana Jones, half Jack Sparrow.

Of course I need the right spot to be adventurous in. In places like South Korea and America when the team is on tour and on a collective mad one, I find that a sprawling megalopolis brings out my need for seclusion. Or to use a football term, it makes me a sulky bastard.

So when one team I played for found itself on the southern tip of Spain for what was called mid-season training camp but which was in reality a massive jolly with a bit of training thrown in, I felt the need to go off and explore the surrounding landscape. Our training ground was set in between the sea and the mountains (as is everything that is not sea or mountains I suppose). I say mountains but I mean pretty big hills. Well, mounds.

One of the hills was noticeably larger than the others and I decided to conquer it. Because it was there. Because I am English and it could be the start of rebuilding the empire, which has been in a transitional phase for some time.

It was hot, well over thirty degrees, when I bravely set off carrying nothing but half the physio room's stock of bottled water and a party barrel of sun cream.

The land was angry that day, my friends, and I never made the summit.

Mountains, even pretty big hills, are like the shoreline as viewed from the stern of a yacht. A visual trick. It seems like you could reach out and touch the land. Try swimming to shore. You'll drown.

I recalled this truth about nine-tenths of the way up the hillock, a climb that had taken me well over three hours since leaving base camp. Then I put my foot on a patch of green shrubbery and promptly disappeared.

The green shrubbery was in fact a cunningly disguised bramble bush. One of the horrible spiky fuckers that countries like Spain grow just to spite tourists who wander off the beaten track. The thing had grown in a big hole and didn't look different in appearance from the greenery all around. I noted this as I shared the hole with the bramble bush.

Climbing that hill in the first place was crazy. Firstly because it was hot. And my usual way of getting to higher ground, the escalator, was not an option. Also, the ascent was dotted with signs all the way up graphically warning trespassers of the threat of explosions and the presence of people with shotguns. These people, though badly drawn, seemed intent on erasing any living thing from the countryside.

I had to get to the top of the hill though, and anyway, I was a professional footballer. Those signs were for other people. Still, at the bottom of that hole I did begin to feel slightly discouraged. There was no way of getting out again without climbing up through the spiky brambles. Or I could wait for the club to launch a large-scale search-and-rescue operation. But suppose they didn't bother. How crushing would that be?

Have you seen the film *Saw*, where one unfortunate captive has to jump into a pit full of hypodermic needles to find a key that will let him out of the door to the room? Me neither. I don't watch shit like that. I live it!

Somebody told me about the movie. If you have seen it, that's what it was like crawling back out of that hole.

Back at the hotel, the dreams of the summit now nothing more than a wistful memory, the physio told me to strip. He knows that usually cheers me up. He walked around me to see if there were any scratches or marks that needed cleaning.

He stopped and laughed. I don't look great from the back but I still felt it was unnecessary. My back, the backs of my legs, the backs of my arms and my regal arse were all dotted with tiny spikes. From certain angles I looked like a porcupine who had learned to walk on two feet. It took the physio and his tweezers two hours and several hundred one-liners to pull most of them out.

The plane ride home was spent sitting in a strange position which favoured my slightly less wounded arse cheek over the other and worried the stewardess no end.

I've never felt the call of the wild again. Adventure is best experienced as nature intended. On PlayStation.

Fines

Physios are a strange breed. They are not really football people. Not really. They have morals and standards of practice and, weirdly, they ask for respect for doing something that most of us players feel they should be doing while down on bended knee.

As such, they have a strange and bastardized version of the fines structure that is prevalent among football ancillary staff. The chef will try to fine you if you don't wash your hands or if you enter his canteen with dirty kit. The kitman will try to fine you if you don't put your socks in the right skip. Ditto your slips (pants), your jumpers, your shorts and your hats and gloves. All of these fines are laid down at the start of the season by the manager and every player signs the fine charter wondering why all the non-playing staff are so fucking OCD about everything.

The rules are written out in black and white and you agree to them because you don't have a choice and because three weeks into the season normal service will be resumed because it is all too much hassle.

The physio lives outside this bubble. He is not a normal football person. His expertise exists beyond football. When football, as my father predicts that it will, finally eats itself, the physio will be able to walk away and become a useful member of society.

He knows this. We know this. Even when a new physio starts at the club fresh and all wet behind the ears from physio school, he knows it too.

They work in their own little room where nobody can question their knowledge because nobody really knows a fucking thing about it. Still, in the spirit of inclusiveness the physio room has its own system of fines too. These rules encompass the following areas, which are of grave concern to mankind:

- Farting in the physio room
- Reading a newspaper or magazine in the physio room
- The wearing of hats in the physio room
- Being on the phone in the physio room
- The wearing of boots in the physio room
- Drinking or eating in the physio room
- Loitering in the physio room (this is a biggie: every physio I've ever worked with has had a 'loitering' fine in place)
- Kicking a ball in the physio room
- Taking all the ice from the ice machine from the physio room
- Leaving the scooper for the ice machine in the ice machine and not on top of the ice machine
- Leaving bags of ice in the sink and not disposing of the ice correctly (global warming, for fuck's sake)
- Oh yeah: swearing in the physio room
- Using the physio's computer/laptop to surf the internet/put music on via YouTube when he's at lunch
- Leaving plaster wrappers and other rubbish on the physio table
- Taking paracetamol, strappings, scissors, nail clippers, in fact anything from the physio room without asking.

Or asking but forgetting to bring them back. For this particular fine I told every physio at every club I ever played for to fucking swivel – you have to remember that some physios are on the take in terms of cash payments, just like the dodgiest managers you can imagine. When your physio rolls up in a brand-new Jag you know it's time to call a team meeting. And we did.

Some of these physios even have their list of 'dos and don'ts' pinned to the door. It's sick really. The thin end of the wedge that is physio fascism.

Then again, they are in the medical profession.

Many happy returns

Behold the player whose birthday it is while he is injured.

Usually a pro player will mark his birthday in the same way that Jesus marks Christmas. He'll get the bumps, and if he's impressionable he might be persuaded to sing a song for the lads, but he never forgets that it is a good day for humanity. So whatever happens he'll always, no matter what, have to bring cakes into the changing room for the lads and also produce another lot of pastries for the staff.

The player who is injured modestly tries to avoid birthdays. No fuss, thanks.

Why? He is of no use to the players, who can't give him the bumps on the training pitch. Instead he becomes a victim of what should be his own party.

Every morning the injured players will see the physio first, at nine a.m. sharp. Thereafter they are generally hooked up to life support machines to treat their ailments. This is when the players strike. Forget the physio issuing fines for fucking about, there are some occasions when anything goes.

The time-honoured tradition is to gather up about six first-team players to run into the physio room, and before the injured player can react, pin him down while a couple of lads wrap clingfilm around him and the bed thus ensuring that he is stuck fast for – well, as long as you like.

Once the first part of the process has been safely concluded, the next phase is to add a little colour to the cheeks of the sick and indigent player. Just take some boot polish and smother his face in it. Apply it thicker than a Geordie lass's make-up on a Friday night oot.

I did once see a pair of shitty slips placed over the face of one of the players. Personally I felt that was taking it too far and I voted against Brexit because I didn't want protection from such war crimes to become a thing of the past. They were my own slips, not the club's.

The all-time best/worst I have seen was a youth-team player who was slight and pigeon-chested and well liked. He was marched from the changing room and clingfilmed to the cross-bar while the first team took pot shots at him from the halfway line. Well, you don't want to kill him. That wouldn't be funny for Christ's sake. Give the poor bastard a chance at least. That's what separates us from the barbarians.

He took it well but always had a phobia afterwards about crossbars and clingfilm.

JANUARY

We've come through the end-of-year madness in one piece and are playing good football. You can sense the general relief around the club. After a couple of fallow seasons and with the arrival of another new manager there had been a submerged fear here that we were just having a short break from bad times and that we might relapse. December is a month when that sort of thing tends to happen, but we have been winning games, keeping players injury-free, and we are in contention. Phew.

Call me Scrooge, I'm just glad Christmas is over and we're now back to some sort of normality. It's humbug-free, January, the most underappreciated of football months. The beauty of it is that it's a much quieter month. We usually play only one match per week. There can be a couple of FA Cup games too, but no European games until February – if you're still alive in Europe that is, which we are.

At a big club, the romance of the FA Cup is that it enables squads to be rotated. Players can be rested, players not playing regularly have a chance and players returning from injury are given an opportunity to get some match play. And if you get knocked out in the third round after fielding a team with seven or eight reserves? Well, then you don't have to play on the weekend of the fourth round. You get an even better break. That's the romance for a lot of us. Win. Win.

Arsenal are having their seasonal crisis. It doesn't always hit them in December or January but it hits them nonetheless. That means there will soon be calls for Arsène Wenger's head to be delivered *sur une assiette*. Thanks for everything, Monsieur Wenger, but adieu.

It's hard to know precisely what the problem is but in my business we all have a theory. Arsenal suffer too many injuries. Year in, year out they have key players unavailable for key matches.

At one stage a few years back an Arsenal fan started a petition to have the entire medical department sacked. Yet Arsenal's medical people/facilities are unlikely to be of an inferior standard to any other top club's.

A couple of seasons ago, when asked about the number of muscle injuries players at Arsenal seemed to suffer, Wenger said, 'Some of them are down to the medication the players take that you don't even know about. Then you realize afterwards that they took this medication and it is not prudent. The liver does not work as well, the toxins do not go as quickly out of the body as they should, and they get tired. If you lose your hair and if you've taken something to make your hair grow, it might not be especially good for the rest of your body.'

I imagine that the medical staff had a collective fit when they read that. Arsenal pointed out afterwards that they had no players on long-term medication, although use of painkillers is standard in most dressing rooms. The medical team had found no concrete link between medications and Arsenal's muscle injury plague.

Raymond Verheijen, the Dutch conditioning guru who has worked with several international sides at World Cups and with big clubs like Barcelona, Bayern Munich and Manchester City, pointed the finger at Wenger and suggested his conditioning training was outdated. 'There is a pattern at Arsenal, and it repeats itself every year. It is a no-brainer.'

A lot of people think that Verheijen has a little bit too much to say for himself and that he does so much finger-pointing that it must be a full-time job for him keeping that index digit of his fully conditioned. Yet he might have a point.

Our traditional method is to take a long summer break, then pile on the punishment during a few weeks of pre-season in a blinkered solution that gives you a short-term level of fitness and conditioning. The quietest time of year in the medical room is generally the final two months of a busy season which seems counter-intuitive to some people. But as games keep coming at players at the rate of two a week their bodies develop precisely the type of hardy conditioning needed for life as a pro.

There is a fine balance to be struck in conditioning work. Doing things the way they always have been done may be to do things the wrong way. Some clubs and many younger managers have begun to appreciate that over the past few years. But the dinosaurs are still out there.

Does a guy like Wenger get to the stage where he sees no reason to do things in any way other than the way things have always been done? Does arrogance prevent these people from looking at other methods?

Arsenal have had the same manager and coaching philosophy for two decades. Is the training too light and not adequately preparing the players for games, rendering them vulnerable to injury both in training and in matches? Or is it too challenging, so that players go into a game fatigued and at risk?

Certainly every year Arsenal tend to have a lot of injuries. Lots of things influence the performance of the team but if you have the full squad to select from you are always in a better place. Arsenal lose key players every campaign and Wenger tends to ignore gaudy distractions like transfer deadline day with a Zen calm. The club has so much potential but they never achieve what they should achieve. At least not any more.

So my gut feeling is that, yes, it has to be down to the training. Same manager for a long time and same problem for a long time. Those things are surely connected.

Arsenal, as gets said every time Wenger is questioned, have been in the Champions League every year since old Noah built the ark. They get games. Plenty of them. They should naturally be hardened from that experience. Yet every year there is a muddy patch that slows them down, a few inexplicable results, and people looking at their injury problems.

We won't know the definitive answer until Wenger goes. He may just be the victim of cruel bad luck on the injury front. Year in and year out. But a lot of people are noticing that since he went on loan to Bournemouth for the season Jack Wilshere has managed a run of games which has been miraculous given that at Arsenal his sick note had to be laminated because he spent most of every season carrying it around with him.

Look at the bigger picture, Arsène. Look in the mirror.

We've just had an FA Cup weekend. We won't be having any more of them this year. Bit of a shocker, Jeff. We were beaten away at a lower-league club.

The FA Cup really is a funny business for big clubs now. It's great to reach Wembley in May. At the end of a long season, it's a good day out. We don't really start thinking about the possibility of getting there till about the fifth round though. Before that the club is pragmatic about things. Champions League qualification is the basic aim every season. Getting knocked out of the FA Cup early is a disappointment but not a disaster. If we had grabbed a late equalizer on Sunday and forced a draw, that would have bothered us. Another game with the stakes ratcheted up a bit by all the hype. Thanks, but no thanks.

We got turned over by a modest League Two side. I enjoy going to those grounds where my own career in football began. There is always a funny mix of welcome and defiance when you get there. It's exciting for them to be entertaining a big club and there is a little bit of pleasure at seeing the Premier League millionaires and their entourage being squeezed into a dressing room the size of a Portakabin before a game.

I don't think we mind the spartan conditions quite as much as the hosts like to think we do, but the 'we're not in Kansas any more' moment came when we got out on to the pitch. The noise was different. The dimensions seemed different. The surface was very different.

All the pitches are pretty good in the Premier League these days. I remember being at Birmingham City once and they had just laid the pitch a few days before. On the wing, when a player put a stud into the ground the earth moved. Literally. The turf would ruck up like a piece of carpet.

It varies massively. Playing an FA Cup game on a really cut-up pitch, as we did on Sunday, is a disadvantage. Again, though, we only have ourselves to blame. We work and train in a perfect environment. Our training pitches, of which we have three that we use in rotation, replicate the heated, knitted-in, floodlit surface we have at the ground. Same grass, same length, same lights, same Desso surface.

A Desso surface, or Desso GrassMaster pitch as the manufacturers like to call it, is a hybrid grass system combining natural grass with artificial fibres. The fibres are injected into the surface to about 8 inches in depth and they occupy about 3 per cent of the pitch. The grass grows and the roots anchor themselves and entwine with the fibres. It creates a better-standard surface and aids the longevity and durability of the grass. Premier League pitches obviously have undersoil heating, drainage and irrigation systems as standard.

All very good, until you go back to playing on good old-fashioned grass and mud.

The more specific and controlled we have made our environment, the less adaptable we have become. If we only play and train on pitches that have been laid like new carpets we are going to have to learn very quickly when we get back out into the real world and the surfaces most football is played on.

It would probably be better to train on different surfaces and pitches, especially in the run-up to a game like last Sunday's, but we all worry about injuries so we end up travelling and hoping for the best.

It was a long journey home on Sunday but a good day out. We enjoyed the welcome, and even when we got our come-uppance we could get a clear sense of what it all meant at a non-corporatized football club that was still local in every way.

We'll be rooting for them to get another good draw.

I've often wondered what, as a medic, you do with a problem like John Terry. He seems like the epitome of the type of player whose heroism brings him to the edge of recklessness when it comes to his own wellbeing. We love those players in England. Terry Butcher with a bloody bandage on his head, Tony Adams, Roy Keane, Bryan Robson. The swashbuckling comic-book heroes.

Terry once finished a game against Manchester United with an ankle injury that saw him travel home on crutches with ten stitches in the wound. For the 2007 League Cup final against Arsenal he declared himself fit to play despite having done his ankle in a Champions League game against Porto on the Wednesday. Then in the final in Cardiff, Terry arrived a split second too late to head a ball away and instead met Abou Diaby's boot. He woke up in an ambulance on the way to hospital and couldn't remember the incident. Neither could he recall his good luck. Arsenal's physio, Gary Lewin, had been tending to the Arsenal keeper Manuel Almunia yards away in the aftermath. Gary realized the gravity of the situation and rushed to attend to the Chelsea skipper. He cleared Terry's windpipe and saved his life.

Still groggy, Terry was out of hospital a couple of hours later and on the flight home, celebrating with his team-mates. He was lucky. Lewin was in the right place at the right time. And with what we know about head injuries now, allowing somebody out of hospital and on to a flight so quickly would never happen.

This week, on behalf of Chelsea, John Terry visited Ryan Mason of Hull in St Mary's Hospital, Paddington. Mason fractured his skull in a league game at Stamford Bridge when he was involved in a clash of heads. When he arrived at St Mary's, surgery was performed. He'll be monitored in hospital for several more days and he is unlikely to play football again this season.

It was interesting to read in the newspapers in the last few days the story of Iain Hume, a Barnsley player who spoke about an elbow by Chris Morgan, then of Sheffield United, in a Championship game in 2008. Hume had been left unconscious. Yet he was sent home that evening and allowed to sleep like a baby all night. He collapsed the following day. It turned out when Hume was taken to hospital that he had a fractured skull and was suffering from internal bleeding. He was left with an eighteen-inch scar running in a horseshoe shape on the side of his head.

What happened to Hume occurred two years after the infamous Petr Cech case in October 2006. Cech has been wearing head protection in games ever since. The John Terry incident at Cardiff came just months after Cech's injury. The lessons of correct treatment of head injuries have been absorbed very slowly.

Medics need to be adamant and strong. Bloodied heroes are

romantic figures. Heroes who are damaged or killed by the game and by their own bravery are tragedies we can avoid.

I like to go along to hospital with a player. There could be something to learn. And spending that time with him builds bridges. You are taking your time to invest in his wellbeing. It's too easy to tell somebody, 'Yeah, you go, and let us know how you get on. I'll be waiting here in my sulk until you get back.'

We are about to be ambushed by another transfer deadline day. This past week I've spent a lot of time liaising with medical staff at other clubs about which players of ours may be sold or loaned. It doesn't look as if there will be too many coming in but it is still a distraction. This year the timing of the January deadline is a complete pain. The window closes on an evening when there is a full slate of fixtures. Teams are on the road or shored up in hotels near their own ground. Getting hold of people has been a nightmare.

There is an enormous difference between medical personnel in clubs in the Premier League and the lower divisions. We are quite well staffed, and if I am taking the load in terms of communicating with clubs before deadline day, I know that somebody else is covering for me at the front line.

I know from experience that life for my colleagues outside the First World that is the Premier League and the Championship is a lot tougher.

My first role in charge of a team was at a League Two club, where I was the only full-time medical person employed for the first-team squad. We had a part-time masseur for games, a fellow physio looking after the youth teams and I saw the club doctor, who was a local GP, only when it was match day or when someone was sick.

At many lower-league clubs, things are still the same. The physio's role is multifaceted. He must be a jack of all trades doing anything from taking sessions to a bit of chiropody and helping out with kit, and sometimes even making sure that the players get some lunch after training. I remember many a trip down to the nearest sandwich shop to buy the squad's lunch. The perk was that they were paying! Things couldn't be more different at the bigger Premier League clubs. Everyone's role is specialized. And if necessary the sandwiches are delivered, and have prawns in them.

It's a far cry from when I first got involved in football, which was almost by accident. I was asked by the head physio of a small club if I could give a hand on Saturday mornings and with the academy one evening a week. I did that for a season while working in private practices and at the end of it was asked to help out covering the professional squad in pre-season. I accepted. After a six-week probation period they offered me a full-time job.

In my first few days I was asked to take the warm-up, and one of the players who loved to have a laugh dropped back and rugby-tackled me. It wasn't quite so much fun for him when I pinned him to the ground as he was struggling to get up. He never crossed me again. I gained a bit of respect that day.

The manager was old-school. He hated injured players and wanted them inconvenienced as much as possible as he suspected they were doing it on purpose to spite him. He made them (and me) stay late in the evenings and come in on days off until they were fit.

The equipment was very basic, and as I didn't have many staff I used machines on the players. Some of those machines were from different countries and God only knows what they did. One of them was like something out of *Star Trek* and it would move automatically up and down a player's injury with a beam of light. No idea what it did but it looked great – and a very effective placebo I'm sure. We had it serviced once and the technician told us it was emitting more radiation than when you have a chest X-ray (and that's quite a lot) . . . so we got rid of it. Which left us with the problem of how to keep those players occupied while we were busy with the others.

I had worked in the NHS where everything is documented and you have to have a good reason for what you do and how you do it. Football was nothing like that. Hardly any staff were writing notes on how they were treating the players, and many of the treatments were carried out not because they were scientifically proven to work, but because they were what the player wanted – which can be a powerful placebo, but that wasn't the reason they did it. Some would only do the treatments they were trained in, or use machines they had available – so whether a player had a sprained ankle, torn groin muscle or bad back, he was given the same treatment!

The size, range of specializations and the expertise within a department now is astonishing. As is the amount of money the medical team costs a club nowadays. A top six Premier League team will spend up to £3 million a year on the department.

I read recently that Coventry City have a budget that size for their entire club.

As a physio at a small club, it used to be that if there was a player with a significant injury history with whom you had worked in the past, your 'inside knowledge' could be very influential. I remember one player who failed a medical at a club the day before deadline. The club asked me about him as I had worked with him before. I told them that the injury was significant but if managed correctly he could play thirty games or more per season. We signed him. And he did. Phew.

> Dear Peaches,
> I recently found out that the little hussy who is the significant midfielder in my life has been seeing a medical guru behind my back. What should I do?
> Devastated Physio

> Dear Dev,
> Try to understand, and don't cause a confrontation. Don't be so possessive. You will be the loser. See what you can learn from this, to maybe make the relationship stronger in the future. Or maybe make yourself stronger. Look, maybe he's just not that into you anyway.
> Peaches

Trust in the department is a big thing. You know that saying, 'The customer is always right'? The player is the customer, but when he comes to the physio department he isn't always right.

Sometimes if he isn't hearing the news he wants to hear he'll start talking to the other players and getting outside advice. Sometimes he might want more treatment than his injury actually merits. So the key thing we have to build is trust. If a player trusts his medical team he will do everything they advise him to do. If, for example, the order is just to rest and take a tablet, he will buy into that. If there is no trust, the player will go off looking for advice elsewhere. This usually happens if they want a second opinion because things aren't progressing as well as they had hoped.

Usually you find out that the second opinion is the same as the advice you gave in the first place. That's OK. You don't crow. My head isn't up my arse. It doesn't have to be me. As long as your player gets fit. Great. If sticking pink tape on your leg makes you feel better, that is good.

Thanks to the immense increase in incomes in the last decade or so, a lot of players started going outside their club environment for treatment – not because they had to but because they could. The guru who extracts a massive wad from a player for some newfangled treatment has no skin in the game, however, and often players come back to us looking for help with the damage that's been done. We don't criticize or scold them. We improve and broaden our knowledge and become more all-encompassing. We find that when players leave us to go to other clubs they often like to come back for an opinion from us when they get injured. It may piss off the other physios but the idea is to improve your own act to the level where that doesn't happen.

When it comes to injuries and sources of repair outside the

club, the attitude of modern players is simple: we'll do whatever we want.

So now we have the phenomenon of the medical guru shadowing the big player, or being available to a group of top players.

These used to be the cures that dared not speak their name, but now players have more power. They used to see their gurus behind the clubs' backs, in hotels and clinics. Now the gurus are part of the furniture. At the club we even have a feng shui consultant to help us arrange them in a way which harmonizes with the environment while they wait around.

When a player arrives with a guru in tow, sometimes we integrate the guru into our lives. Just because a guru is different doesn't mean that the guru is a charlatan. Sometimes when a player wants to visit a guru we will travel along as chaperones. We make sure nobody gets hurt. Sometimes we learn something useful and the skills become a beneficial part of our philosophy.

This flexibility and acceptance is a soft skill that medics and managers have to learn. We have to communicate. We have to be open. We have to accept that sometimes these people actually help. Who am I to say they are wrong? I just make sure the player is safe and that the guru isn't going to imperil that. I try to be part of the process. I try to be educated by the process. Sometimes we are scared of what these gurus are doing in case they make us feel incompetent.

On the other hand, a lot of gurus take advantage. They offer ridiculous treatments to desperate players. A seriously injured player will do anything.

You see, players trust other players. If one player says to another player, 'Look, this guy makes you walk like a duck and it's amazing, my ankle healed up in three weeks, you should definitely go to him with your hamstring,' the second player is always impressed. Now usually the first player's ankle would have healed up in three weeks anyway, and even if walking like a duck helped, who knows what this particular guru knows about hamstrings?

You try to have adult conversations with the player about the process. And at the same time you have to accept that for modern players recovery options don't begin and end at the club medical room.

Hans-Wilhelm Müller-Wohlfahrt has become a multi-millionaire partly through injecting Actovegin (derived from calves' blood) into patients at his Munich clinic. His use of homeopathic medicine to treat players is controversial but Healing Hans has treated everybody from Paula Radcliffe, José María Olazábal, Boris Becker, Michael Owen, Darren Gough and Usain Bolt through to His Holiness Bono (Bono no longer performs 'I Still Haven't Found What I'm Looking For' since having severe compression of the sciatic nerve cured). Asked to solve the problem of English cricketer Michael Vaughan's recurrent knee injury, Hans returned to the farmyard to muster up an injection of Hyalart, a gel-like mixture formed from crushing the fleshy pink comb from a cockerel's head. Do not try that at home, by the way.

In the summer of 2012, Peter MacDonald of St Johnstone in Scotland had an epidural and got pin-cushioned with more than fifty injections of goats' blood by Müller-Wohlfahrt.

MacDonald had hamstring problems. He is still playing at the age of thirty-seven.

The benefits of Actovegin have never been peer-reviewed, i.e. properly scientifically proven. As far as I can tell the substance is not approved in the US, but it is not on the World Anti-Doping Agency's list of banned substances even though Travis Tygart, the head of the United States Anti-Doping Agency (USADA), has called Actovegin injections a 'Frankenstein-type experiment'.

Nevertheless, players will fly to Munich at the drop of a hat if they think it will make them better.

In fact they will go anywhere.

In November 2009, when Robin van Persie was carried off on a stretcher screaming in agony after just ten minutes of Holland's international with Italy, his season seemed as good as over. The first word that Arsène Wenger received that night was that the player's ankle was likely to be fractured so the Arsenal manager approached the remainder of the weekend in a dark mood. At Arsenal they are used to bad injury news and they assumed that van Persie was out for the rest of the campaign.

Van Persie thought differently. He announced that he was off to Belgrade to get some placenta treatment. His damaged ligaments would be healed in a jiffy, he assured his boss. And so the little-known Mariana Kovacevic became a Premier League curiosity for a while.

There is nothing new under the sun in football though. The Dutch striker had learned of the treatment on the grapevine from his Dutch team-mate Orlando Engelaar, who had been clued in to Kovacevic's unorthodox methods by Serbian team-mate Danko Lazović. Van Persie was initially quoted as having been pleased with the treatment, but it soon became clear that it had not worked. The torn ankle ligaments kept him out of football for the rest of the season.

Placenta injections may have sounded like a new fad but Rafa Benítez in his time at Liverpool was a believer, and Manchester City also booked players in. Guys like Nigel de Jong, Vincent Kompany, Fábio Aurélio, Yossi Benayoun and Glen Johnson all made the trip to see the Serbian healer. Not long after van Persie went, Frank Lampard followed with Chelsea club doctor Bryan English in tow, although the London club insisted that Lampard's trip was solely to receive deep massage. Some years later, while playing for Atlético Madrid, Diego Costa flew to Belgrade for treatment with the approval of Diego Simeone.

Kovacevic's healing technique involved massaging horse placenta deep into damaged tissue. The cells within the placenta were alleged to speed up the healing process. Once the placenta had been rubbed deep into the flesh, electrical equipment would be attached to the leg and the skin around ligaments and muscles. The stimulation improved the chances of the medicine reaching the various places of injury, apparently.

Wenger's reaction to his star striker heading off to Belgrade to have some equine placenta injected into him was pretty much what my own would have been. 'I am not a fan but also I am not a doctor,' Wenger said. 'Van Persie said he wanted to go, so I asked my medical people if there was any danger. They said no, so I let him go. But I've never seen anybody with a muscle problem [be fit] short of twenty-one days, never seen anyone go there and five days later he plays.'

There is a German doctor in Munich, Dr Ulrike Muschaweck, who specializes exclusively in hernias of the abdominal wall and groin region. Her technique is known as the Munich Repair. The claim is that players who go for this repair are back playing within a week. I've known players who had her procedure and it hasn't worked, but who haven't been back or haven't contacted her, so for all I know she may think they are better.

Jamie Redknapp has been quoted as saying that he even went to an osteopath who wanted to take his wisdom teeth out to treat his knee injury.

Then there is the Spanish love of treatment called epi, which is an electronic acupuncture. They swear by it. It's tempting to ask, but if it is so good, how come it is only used in Spain? That is no help though. All I hear about it is it's bloody painful and fries tissue.

In the UK we have made our own contribution to this rich tapestry – when Glenn Hoddle introduced us to the world of Eileen Drewery.

Some people go to soft-tissue therapists or deep-tissue masseurs who stick their thumbs in and rip the living daylights out of the area. This appeals greatly to the player who feels that if there is pain there must be gain. The problem, as I said earlier, is that these external guys have no skin in the game. If it doesn't work they shrug their shoulders and say you need to go back and talk to your club physio. This always works, but it's not working on you. So sorry. Ask the club to take another look. Pay at reception on your way out. Thank you! So the problem comes back to the club. The player walks in a little sheepishly and we can't just tell him to go back to that quack who they thought was Jesus a few weeks ago. We have to help. We have to find the solution. We can't discharge our players and send them back to the GP, unlike in the NHS.

That's not to say that medical departments at clubs don't pass players on to external bodies for treatments. It's just that clubs are old-fashioned about choosing the hands they will place their players in. They are particular about who they trust.

We know what we will get with a surgeon, for example. He or she will cut the player open, fix what is broken and stitch him up again. So we put the player into their hands because their methods are tried and tested and we understand them.

The problem is that players (despite what you might think) generally are gullible and good-natured. If a player gets injured and he gets a call or a text from a player he respects – for, say, his goalscoring prowess – he's just as likely to believe that player when he tries to diagnose him or recommends some outlandish new process.

In his autobiography, Niall Quinn tells a story about injuring his knee when he was playing at Manchester City. Quinn got a call from Alan Shearer, whom he had never met. Shearer recommended a surgeon. Quinn, who is obviously a very sensible man, went straight to the surgeon Shearer had named, giving a swerve to Manchester City's own surgeon. After the surgery, as luck would have it, septicaemia set in. These things happen. What struck a chord with me, though, was Quinn's account of calling Eamonn Salmon, the physio at City, to tell him that he'd had his surgery done elsewhere: 'I've never heard a man have a coronary down the phone line before. Eamonn goes into denial. He says I'm winding him up. He tells me that he will be sacked. He goes back to his coronary.'

I have been that soldier.

Some surgeons come and go in fads, like one-hit wonders. There used to be a guy in Colorado, Richard Steadman. He did everybody's knees. He was hugely popular. His clinic has passed on to a younger generation and is still very good. There was a time when everybody went there, but then the craze moved on somewhere else. There are a few guys who are very good at what they do, a few specialists the proven quality of whose work makes them worth the journey.

But just because a guy is famous doesn't mean he is right for you in terms of specialization. Remember, once the knife slices into you there is no reset button. I have had players who have been adamant that they want surgery with a particular surgeon and they come back and that surgeon has been overzealous or has performed an inappropriate operation. The player knows he has screwed up by going against the advice of the club. Sometimes the agent or his parents have nudged him.

I understand that for foreign players in particular, they might want to go home and get cured in an environment they are familiar with. What we tend to do is find out who the best French guy is if a French player wants to go home for surgery, and so on. When you have a multicultural club you cannot have a problem with a French player wanting a French surgeon. Our problem is the player being seen by just *any* French surgeon. So we buy into the process a bit and recommend particular practitioners. We understand that Andy Williams and Jonathan Webb, both knee surgeons in the UK, are excellent, but if a

Spanish player busts his knee we also understand that he will probably want to see Ramón Cugat in Barcelona, as Cugat sees all the Barça and Real players.

The terrain may be pitted and muddied, but my task remains the same – to lead my players safely to the other side.

We're turning the corner into February. We have basically the same squad that we started the year with and we are getting back to the two-games-a-week rhythm which we will sustain right till the end, I hope. We are nicely placed and have the knockout stages of the Champions League to look forward to.

From now on the team will scarcely train at all. It will be game, recovery session next day, some light work the day before the following match, and then play again. We like where we are at. As a club, that is the pace we have been built to operate at. There is no sense of adventure or trepidation. Let's just get the work done.

I keep telling people that I'm not a big fan of football, but I do like this time of the year. Serious games and a little adrenalin rush from the pressure on the medical room as we keep patching them up and putting them back out there.

TSF: Second Opinion

Beware the creature of habit

A kid I used to look after in my fledgling agency came to me because the agent he was with, like so many of them, only cared about the players who had made it to the big time. And by 'big time' I mean that time when the agent could get north of £100K for doing a deal with a club for his player.

Young players are gobbled up into the big agencies with the promise of free boots. Believe me, this still works. Boots cost more than £150 a throw these days and some of these kids earn less than that a week, particularly in the lower leagues.

So when this kid says to his agent, 'Mister, I need boots,' the agent duly obliges. Unfortunately for the kid, the agent is a tight fuck. Who knew?

He sends four pairs of boots addressed to the kid at the club. Two pairs of moulded and two pairs of studs, the industry standard for freebies. The boots turn up. The kid is going to look like the dog's.

'My boots are here!' he announces. All the other kids are sick jealous. He opens the first box and there is nervous laughter. The agent has sent boots all right. They have the name of Arsenal full-back Carl Jenkinson stitched into the leather along one side, together with an English flag, beautifully embroidered underneath. The kid is Irish.

Some mistake surely, he says. (Did I mention that he was Irish?)

He opens the next box, and the next. All the same. Carl Jenkinson's boots.

This happened.

Boots were the bane of my footballing life. I would find a pair that I loved. They'd fit me perfectly. I would have married those boots if I had been allowed. I would have at least entered into a civil partnership. They completed me.

Then the manufacturer would change them or discontinue them. This may come as a shock but lots of players trawl eBay for the boots they love after they have been changed or discontinued because footballers are creatures of habit. I've done it myself. And for a donation of just £5 a month you can help to end the suffering of so many millionaire footballers.

Footwear is obviously a massive part of the game. I believe that in this regard, whatever the player wants he should be given. Whatever makes him feel more comfortable and whatever makes him play better is what he should have. If he has a superstition about only wearing a long top or cutting the sleeves off his gear, fucking let him. If he doesn't want his boot boy to clean his boots because he likes the worn-in feeling then fucking don't let the boot boy clean them. Fire the boot boy.

One physio I worked with was ahead of the curve in this respect. He saw the advantages. I have been fined for wearing 'inappropriate footwear' in the gym. It was a pair of Nike Rifts. Not exactly ideal for lifting weights, but then again, who gives a fuck? I liked them, they were comfortable. My next physio cottoned on to this. He called the Rifts 'cosmetic footwear'. He had my back, he let me wear them.

The players, footwear philistines to a man, took the piss at first.

'If he plays well on Saturday and we win then he can wear clogs for all I care.'

Wrong. But quite right too.

The England interview

One senior physio I am fortunate enough to know once applied for the England physio job.

Now this physio friend isn't quite the best in the business. That honour belongs to the man writing this book with me. But he is a close second. Personal honours, titles, Champions League nights, you name it. Been there, done that, and tried to look interested in the football too.

He is less than enamoured with football and its politics so he asks me for my input when it comes to job prospects. He had been invited to apply for the England post and he didn't know what to do.

'Go for it,' I said.

Obviously it would be very good for his medical career if he could inadvertently become a source for gossip from the England camp.

So he threw his cap into the ring.

As it turned out, the FA interview was a gusher of good anecdotes. My friend gave all the right answers but came away with hundreds of questions.

The interview was conducted over a week at St George's Park, England's new training headquarters set in the epicentre of world football that is Burton-on-Trent. My friend still had a busy day job with one of the best clubs in the country. He couldn't afford to stay in the deserted St George's Park hotel, so he commuted instead. Two hours up and two hours back, every day.

He was in confident mood. If they headhunt you then you know you are in with a chance.

The interview was to be a theoretical and practical mix. Highlights of the process included stepping into the cavernous grotto that the FA believes is a modern gym (they think that having every single piece of gym equipment ever invented qualifies the grotto as 'state of the art'). My friend was told that he would have to conduct a session with some players.

At the far end were two basketball players who were wheelchair-bound. These were the players with whom he was to perform. My friend is a lovely man and a wonderful physio and I have no doubt that had he been given the time he would have had both of the lads slam-dunking. As it was, he had to scrap the football session he had in his head and do some coaching work with these two guys.

As a football physio my mate had seen a lot of bad injuries but he had never experienced a tragedy like two players becoming wheelchair-bound and only interested in playing basketball.

Perhaps, he thought, this is what is wrong with English football at international level. Too much training and thinking like wheelchair basketball players.

On day two, the FA decided to sell itself to the candidates. My physio friend was shown 'the master plan'. The plan was the FA's attempt to give itself the kiss of life.

I've seen the chart. It's huge. It's as if you took a whole school's worth of primary-school kids and asked them to take out their rulers and pencils and prepare tables that showed what subjects they would be studying and when over the coming year. It had to be a table that made their parents say, perhaps you should go out to play more often?

The FA plan had little gaily coloured boxes all over it. Each one of those boxes related to a job that was either taken (yellow), or in the process of being filled (green), or which was vacant (pink). This interview happened two months before Euro 2016. The plan was pretty much a sea of pink. To fill all the pink boxes in time for Euro 2016 would have required mass conscription not interview processes.

I'd never seen so many jobs on offer. The sheer number of pink boxes simply wiped out the immigration problem. There were jobs for everybody. And all in the FA. I decided that if the FA were going to fill all those posts then I was going to invest serious money in the blazer industry. It was going to be boom time for blazer makers. If you wanted a job at the FA prior to Euro 2016 then you could have walked into Wembley Stadium, chucked a dart blindfolded at a massive spreadsheet, and the chances are that the FA would have offered you the head of youth development gig if that's where your arrow landed.

My favourite part of his story resulted in some total and utter car-crash comedy inspired, I imagine, by Basil Fawlty.

'OK,' said the interviewer, 'you're going to interview the head physio of Manchester United today. He's in this room.'

'Where?'

'There.'

'That is not the head physio of Manchester United. I know the head physio of Manchester United. That is not him.'

'Well, no,' said the FA man. 'This man is an actor. He is going to play the part of the head physio of Manchester United. He is angry because Wayne Rooney has been sent back from England duty injured.'

Now this was an interesting scenario. Millions of pounds of valuable player flesh at stake. You think that transfer windows are crazy periods of financial excess? You should see what insurance companies deal with daily over the course of a year. Every year.

A player coming back from international duty injured is an

insurance company's nightmare. Clubs pay millions of pounds out to insure against such an outcome and the FA contribute too. A player returning from international duty with a sore hamstring is one thing; a player coming back with a broken leg is quite another. As I write, the case of Séamus Coleman and Ireland makes the point exactly. Séamus got his leg broken in two places playing for Ireland against Wales. He will miss the best part of a year. Everton won't be paying his wages for that time, FIFA will. And many hundreds of pages of forms will be shuffled around to make that happen.

When I watch international football I never feel that it has the intensity of domestic football. Insurance is a part of that.

'He wasn't injured when we sent him,' said the actor.

'Yes he was,' said my friend. 'Where are his medical records?'

Every physio should send through an up-to-date record of every player's injuries for exactly this purpose. Insurance contingencies.

'I haven't got them,' said the actor. 'Why did you play him?'

'He said he had a tight groin. We'd never have played him if we had the medical records though,' my friend countered.

'Well you must be able to tell if he was injured?'

'He complained of some slight discomfort in the area. He wanted to play. If you thought otherwise you would have sent his records on.'

When players are called up for England but don't play it is usually because there has been an insurance claim before the match. It is that innocuous. In the last ten years, as money has flooded into the game, the relationships between club and country have deteriorated. And that is mainly because of insurance claims and poor communications.

My physio friend said that the fake Manchester United employee was as good if not better than the real thing when it came to having a row. He said that he'd fully researched his stuff and he seemed incredulous that Rooney should have been sent back from England duty with an injury.

Afterwards, my friend asked the actor if he'd had any idea what he was saying. 'Not a clue,' said the actor.

By day three my physio friend was wondering what he had done to deserve a shot at the England job. Something bad in a previous life perhaps. He'd have to ask Glenn Hoddle.

On day four, the mayhem all but petered out. My physio friend had given a good account of himself and kept a straight face throughout.

As with all these processes, the final phase was the delicate chat about money.

'What is your present annual wage, Mr Physio?'

'£150,000 per annum.'

'Uhhh . . . really?'

'Is there a problem?'

'Wow. Well this job pays £75,000 per annum. But it is the FA. This is England. So yes, 75K.'

And all the blazers you can eat.

Physician, heal thyself

In every physio room in world football there are the same laminated posters of the physical marvel that is the human body. Not my body, but a similarly idealized one.

This has led to a problem. Players who imagine they are

smarter than they actually are (a pretty low bar in many cases) think that they know about lots of stuff other than football. They have begun to diagnose their own injuries.

Just wait until they discover that the internet isn't behind the goals on a pitch in Milan.

A little knowledge is a dangerous thing and pisses off every physio in every club in every league in the world. Physios genuinely believe that a minimum of four years of full-time education makes them more qualified than a footballer who has looked at a poster.

In the worst cases, the players actually believe that they are graciously imparting knowledge to the physio. They do this because only they can feel the exact pain in their bodies. They know this pain is probably uncharted waters for most medical professionals so they helpfully look at the poster to locate the relevant part of the body and its medical name.

'Look, mate, I don't want to tell you your job but it feels to me like a haematoma, probably of the inguinal type but possibly also femoral. I think we'll have to face up to a herniorrhaphy sooner rather than later.'

'Yada yada yada. Show me again where it is. This blister? Is that what you mean?'

Whenever I heard talk like this I liked to wind up these players by convincing them that they had multiple sclerosis or something worse.

'Ohhh – seriously mate?' (And then look away as if stricken.)

'What, mate? What do you think it is? Tell me for fuck's sake.'

'Look, I didn't tell you this, and wait till you get the test results back before you panic, but last time I heard about those symptoms the guy was dead within three weeks. But, look, I could be wrong. And he was a lot younger than you so that might make a difference. Wait for the test results.'

'Shit. I'm scared, mate.'

'Did they do the brain scan yet?'

'No, why? Would I need a brain scan? Oh fuck.'

'Doesn't matter. Forget I mentioned anything about the brain scan. It was nothing.'

The players who are most desperate to diagnose their own injuries are the same ones who will listen to any old wino who offers a grave opinion on the same injury. Hours of fun.

Conversely, there are the wishful thinkers, distant cousins of the catastrophists. They hobble in off the training ground and breezily announce to the physio that they most definitely have tweaked a hamstring. They are adamant about this because they know if they wish hard enough and it is actually a hamstring they'll be able to play at the weekend.

It's actually a grade one injury and it needs treatment and anything up to a week out.

The wishful thinker won't hear of it. No, I've had it before. Just a tweak of the old hammer, mate. See, it's the thing that runs up here. I'd know the feeling any time. Wasn't even going to mention it but I know what you're like, all professional and shit.

So they go through the charade of a scan and a diagnosis with an expert. Lo and behold, it is a grade one hamstring injury and requires a week on the sidelines. The player is pissed off. The physio is anything but smug. Just exasperated.

I had no idea what the fuck my injuries were unless it was blatantly obvious. That time when I was beheaded was a no-brainer, for instance. A player knows when he's properly pulled his hamstring or done himself serious damage. But defer to the experts. That's what they're there for. I can't read the Latin on a poster of the human body any more than a top physio ever needs to refer to it.

Actually, you have to wonder who the laminated posters bursting with Latin names of the human body are actually for, don't you?

Physios are just asking for it really. Football is nothing if not keeping up with appearances and even the medics aren't above it.

Hiding injuries

I hated players who hid their injuries.

First rule of hidden injury club? Talk about hidden injury club. Most players who hide injuries want people to know that they're hiding their injuries. They want to tell you and make you complicit.

My very first professional club had a captain who thrived on the Friday-night rumour that appeared every week in the local rag: 'Talisman a doubt for clash'.

That was Mick Talisman. Overrated and full of bullshit.

Every Thursday he would throw a tiny, insignificant injury into the mix and the exasperated physio would have to tell the manager and the manager would have to tell the PR flack who would have to tell the hungry media who desisted from their epic investigations into society's ills to run with the Talisman crisis. If it bleeds, it leads. If it's a strain, it makes the back page yet again.

Every week without fail. Breaking news. And every Saturday, without fail, the miracle of the resurrection. Our captain would lead us out to a rapturous ovation.

'Oh thank God, thank Allah, he is risen!'

'There's only one Mickey Talisman, one . . .'

Crowd beside themselves every fucking week. Being beside themselves actually doubled the attendance.

I used to ask the physio why he put up with this bullshit. 'It makes him play better' was the answer. Big lesson. Give the players what they want and be happy in thine own self.

To be honest, that is harder to achieve than a 50-yard free kick against Gianluigi Buffon.

Not that I've tried either.

FEBRUARY

I'm sparing a thought for two strikers today: Callum Wilson of Bournemouth and Danny Ings of Liverpool. Ings made his debut for Liverpool on 29 August 2015. A few weeks later, in mid-October, in his first training session with new boss Jürgen Klopp, Ings suffered an anterior cruciate ligament injury in his left knee. The injury seemed to rule him out for the remainder of that season. Ings returned sooner than anticipated though and made a substitute appearance in the final game of last season.

He would have been forgiven back then for thinking that he had the summer to work on his conditioning. He could look forward to August when his career at Liverpool would begin again. And so it happened. But in late October the news broke that he had sustained impact damage to his right knee in a League Cup match with Spurs. Diagnosis? Another spell on the sidelines for up to nine months. He needed an operation in London on his cartilage.

Then just yesterday Callum Wilson suffered his second devastating anterior cruciate knee ligament injury in the space of just sixteen months and will miss at least the rest of this season. During training, he ruptured the ACL of his left knee. He had suffered the same injury on his right knee in September 2015.

The knee is a minefield for a footballer and more often than not it is the anterior cruciate ligament that explodes. It is situated inside your knee going from the front of the shin bone (tibia) to the back of the thigh bone (femur) and basically stops the shin bone from moving forward when you twist and turn on the knee. The ACL is one of the most dreaded of all football injuries, and the initial agony endured by the player is painful to witness.

A club can expect at least one ACL explosion per squad per season so implementing strategies to prevent them from happening can be time well spent. These can entail anything from simply ensuring players fully recover between games and are not playing while fatigued to working on their jumping and hopping techniques (plyometric training).

There was a time when just about the worst news you could break to a player was that his anterior cruciate had busted. It was a career-defining moment. Now it is just a setback. The last ACL I treated, the player was match-fit again in less than four months. Back in the day we would never have dreamed of getting a player back in that short a stretch of time. It used to take about a year. This quick return does come with an element of risk of re-injury (even of the other knee), but then we are in a high-risk business. The ACL remains a cruel injury to suffer but the tunnel is shorter now. A rehabbing player can see the light from quite early on.

ACL surgery and rehabilitation have come a long way since

the early 1990s when Paul Gascoigne infamously injured his in the FA Cup final tackling Gary Charles. He was out for *sixteen* months. Nowadays that recovery period has been whittled down to a maximum of six months as the footballer will need an operation to replace the ligament with a grafted tendon, usually taken from their hamstring or the tendon on the front of their knee. Some surgeons used to use artificial grafts, but these weren't very robust and tended to re-tear. Work is in progress to see if they can be repaired (i.e. by sewing up what remains) rather than reconstructed (replacing the whole lot). The reconstructed graft is in fact strong enough to cope with the stresses of football at three and a half months but the strength and control of the knee takes longer to fully recondition. Some players have complications such as infection after surgery, too, which can set them back for months.

The period following reconstruction can be long and painful for players, both physically and mentally, and keeping the rehab varied and interesting is one of the physio's main challenges. We sometimes ship our players out to specialist clinics in the UK such as Isokinetics, or to the United States, Qatar or France, just to break up the monotony of the process.

It's a harsh reality that when a treatment room is populated by players who have a chance of making the next game and one player with a long-term injury, such as an ACL victim, it is the latter who usually suffers. The long-term injury can easily get put to the back of the queue as it is not seen as the priority. This can be demoralizing. The biggest clubs have more than enough staff and facilities to avoid this, but even departments like ours are better geared for dealing with short-term priorities than taking time with an ACL rehab. Sometimes we just don't *have* the time.

Not all sportspeople need to have surgery after rupturing their ACL. The decision on whether or not to operate will depend on their level of activity and the type of sport they play. As the ACL is essentially a supporting strut that stabilizes the knee when you twist and turn, if you participate in a sport where you run in straight lines or your body weight is already supported – by a bike, for instance – as long as you regain full knee flexibility and undertake a thorough strengthening and reconditioning programme, you won't need to go under the knife and you'll be able to take up your sport again sooner and with no long-term implications. These sportspeople are known as copers. In football, though, you need a stable knee and that usually means an intact ACL.

Some players are ACL-deficient copers without realizing. I had one player who had an MRI scan for an unrelated problem only to discover that his ACL was ruptured. He had played every game for the past two years with no problems and only then recalled that a year ago his knee had felt a bit stiff but he'd shrugged it off and carried on.

That's no comfort to Ings or Wilson as they start once again on the lower slopes of a long and cruelly familiar climb.

One of the key elements in helping a player recover from long-term injury is motivating them to commit to what can be a long, tough process. That's why good managers keep injured players involved in the team, making them go to team meetings and watch training. This involvement is especially important if the injured player is a senior member of the squad who wields a lot of influence. Sometimes that means that if there is a training session, we have nothing to do, as all the injured players are out there watching. This is a win-win as I get a break and the player feels bonded to squad and team.

Too many times I've seen managers ostracize crocked players. They see injury as failure and don't realize how much it hurts a player to be dismissed as a dead man limping. Invariably, when they are fit and well again the manager is all over them like a cheap spray tan. Those players realize deep down that there will be a time when they are useful again, but all too soon they feel that they are just pieces of meat and they want out. This is how relationships break down.

When you hear of managers 'losing the dressing room', sometimes there is a side to the story other than player petulance. If enough players have had bad experiences with clubs and managers they learn to pretty much look after themselves, even if they say all the right things on TV and do a lot of inspirational shouting in pre-match huddles.

Serious injury is like a grieving process. Grief manifests itself differently of course from person to person. We had a young lad in his early twenties miss the entirety of last season. He was fantastic all the way through. Jovial, happy, accepting of what had happened. That's life, he'd say. Shit happens. I have to make the best of it. Other players, they can't believe it. They are in denial. Over time, they accept the process. Then they get back and find it tough. There's lingering pain, they don't move the same way, and it all seems very slow and frustrating.

It's a horrible thing as a physio to have to tell a player that his career is over. Sometimes that moment comes after a catastrophic injury. It's even worse if you have worked for over a year with a player and every time you show him that the dawn is near, his body breaks down again. Rehab is so hard and tough and lonely that giving them that bad news is rough. The younger the player, the worse the process feels.

The interesting thing is that stats show that you do need to get back quickly when you suffer an injury. The longer you are out for, the less chance you have of playing again, much less returning to the same level. So it is important for us in the medical room to stay positive and do everything we can to get them back as quickly and safely as possible.

The general rule of thumb, especially with younger players, is to ramp up their training sessions gradually. The pace and intensity are less at the outset which gives them time to build the confidence and conditioning to cope with the highest level. They feel like they are getting there. They are improving. They have objective markers: I am better than a week ago; I am doing so much more than I was last month. This is what we are going to achieve, we tell them. We show them how things are broken down. It gives them motivation. If a player has an ACL injury, you're hoping that in three months he'll be running, but between months two and four we need to get him strong and conditioned. In those last two months you'll do a lot of fieldwork with him, then get him into some training – getting the coaches involved. A goalie can do some handling quite early on, keep his hand-to-eye coordination sharp, but no running or jumping or diving.

Players rarely vocalize fear of their skills deserting them, but it must cross their minds. As a physio you are by nature realistic but you err on the side of optimism at all times. You may be able to reduce the recovery period a little bit. You could easily cover yourself by saying somebody will be out for a year, but if you say nine months, that is more achievable and the player will work harder towards that goal. If you go the other way and say you could be out for a year and a half, that player will be demotivated.

A breakdown during rehab is difficult. The player invariably sees it as a failure. To be honest, so does the physio. But you have to deal with it. Life is shit. It isn't fair. These things happen if you are pushing the limits to try to get somebody back quickly; you may occasionally overcook it and someone will break down. Luckily I haven't had too many players who have had a catastrophic breakdown. Even, say, an ACL reconstruction. Some players re-rupture; a high percentage rupture the other knee. It happens. A player gets back from one knee and within a year they do the other one. We can't do a lot about it. Just get you going and continue to work on it.

For us right now, life continues to be good, hovering as we are in Champions League territory around the top of the table. Poor Crystal Palace got tonked on Saturday by their relegation rivals Sunderland. The Palace fans were incensed by what they saw. Chants of 'You're not fit to wear the shirt' rocked Selhurst Park, and one player was confronted on the field by a fan at half-time. Not good. The word seeping out afterwards was that Palace were cancelling a trip to Dubai as a sign that they recognized the gravity of the situation. Later in the week the message changed slightly. They hadn't even got around to booking the Dubai trip anyway. It was never a big deal. Not with everything so fraught.

I wonder about the wisdom of these trips.

A few years back Manchester City flew their galácticos to the UAE for a short break and arrived back just nineteen hours before a cup tie with Middlesbrough. City lost 2-0.

A lot of people have asked me about this. Should they not have flown back earlier? Should they have gone at all? Should they really have played a friendly against Hamburg while they were over there? Let's face it, it was little more than a promotional visit for the club's ever-generous Abu Dhabi backers.

You can look at this both ways. It was something new, different, a fly-away pick-me-up in the sun when the fixtures allowed it. A change is as good as a rest, sort of thing. But it comes at a price. Firstly, travelling to Dubai is no novelty for the modern player. Secondly, you head to that part of the world and it's a new climate – at least twenty degrees warmer than the usually miserable Manchester weather, and all that dry heat! The body needs time to adjust. Thirdly, as the former Arsenal player Martin Keown has suggested, in the middle of the season players are often in greater need of time *away* from each other and the manager than they are of a week of forced bonding. Take some players anywhere and all they will do is look at their mobile phones anyway.

Of course, these trips are short. Five to seven days at best. So just as the body is adjusting to the different environment out there . . . it's time to come home again. You pack your players on to a long flight and hope that they swiftly readjust to English weather.

Palace may have been chastened a bit, but I notice that during the next FA Cup weekend Sunderland, Liverpool, West

Ham, Stoke and Everton, and possibly others, will all be away. David Moyes is taking his struggling Sunderland side to New York for a break. He says that the weather over there will make his players feel like they are in Dubai when they come back to the temperate north-east. Or maybe a week away from home will make them feel that there are worse things in life than relegation.

For me, trips to the USA carry more potential for disruption than trips to Dubai. The time difference is greater. Some players handle that easily because, well, some players adapt to travel better than others do. Travelling is a skill in itself – sleeping in different hotels, coping with jet lag, etc. Players who struggle with travel will inevitably fare worse if they have had a few late nights bookended by long flights into different time zones.

As a physio, of course, the nightmare of having any team taking a break during the winter in New York is that some of them might get the bright idea to go ice skating on the rink at the Rockefeller Center. In 2015, when he was at Southampton, Ronald Koeman took his squad to Switzerland on one of these mid-season breaks. They skied and played ice hockey using muscle groups they wouldn't use in the course of a football season. Nobody got injured, but still – tut-tut. Southampton only won one of their last six games in the league that season.

I remember one of our mid-season trips to a complex in Portugal when we went for a team walk around a lake and a few players thought it would be a great idea to go waterskiing. The persuasive captain spoke to the manager and swore they were all competent at it. One sprained medial collateral ligament, a sprained wrist and even a bout of gastroenteritis from imbibing the stagnant water – great idea!

Last year Claudio Ranieri gave the Leicester City players a week off after they got knocked out of the FA Cup. They were told to go away and forget about football and spend time with wives, friends and loved ones. For players who spend so much time away from home that was a genuine treat. A few of them flew to Dubai as a group with their partners and kids. They ended up staying in the same hotel as Sunderland, who were there on a training break.

'It was a great idea,' said Jamie Vardy. 'I remember sitting on a sun lounger and in the same hotel Sunderland were there, running up and down the beach doing fitness. For me to be relaxing while they were doing the training was quite nice.'

This year, Jürgen Klopp is taking Liverpool down to La Manga for what he calls a mini pre-season. As a physio looking at a team already showing a few signs of tiredness, I think the Ranieri method would suit Liverpool better.

Maybe that's why I've never been asked to manage though.

A few pages back I mentioned the Spanish surgeon Ramón Cugat. Cugat's background is interesting. Since the mid-sixties he has worked with a remarkable organization called Mutualitat Catalana de Futbolistes (MCF). In Spain all levels of soccer player are highly regarded, and for the last eighty years the MCF has ensured the continuing health of non-professionals through-out Catalunya. All active, federated players in the country need to have insurance, and in Catalunya the MCF, a non-profit organization, provides cover for players too. 'The mission is to treat soccer players' injuries and to accompany the player to the safe return to soccer,' Cugat has said. Nearly all the big names in orthopaedic surgery offer their services to the MCF. In our business, it is the medical equivalent of a supergroup.

Barcelona's MCF reference centre comprises four teams involving fourteen orthopaedic surgeons and sports medicine specialists with rehabilitation, diagnostic imaging and sonography departments. Every weekend roughly 1,600 clubs play 4,000 matches and the wounded wash up in the MCF centres which treat every conceivable sort of injury so long as it occurred while playing or training for football.

The MCF staff get to see a huge number of very specific sports pathologies. They track players through their careers. Apart from developing an incredible expertise with the common-or-garden footballing injuries, they also see problems that professionals at top clubs seldom see because of the low volume of patient traffic.

Cugat operates on twenty to thirty players a week. The MCF hosts up to a dozen visiting fellows a year, generously allowing their knowledge to spread.

I love this idea.

If I was looking after physios on a national level I would create mentorships. A Premier League or Championship physio would mentor the staff at a lower-league club which was geographically close. Crawley Town could use Brighton, for example. Aldershot could use Chelsea. Swindon could use Reading, just down the M4. Scunthorpe might look west towards Leeds, or further, to Manchester or Liverpool. Just to have a link. Just to have somebody to bounce ideas off, to create an environment of consultation, mutual help and advice with problem cases.

This would mean physios at lower levels being supported all the way through. And it is lonely down in the lower leagues. Imagine working at Plymouth, miles away from anybody. It must be hard and isolating. You are on your own. It wouldn't take much to change that.

Let's spread the knowledge and experience.

I've been reading about how Under Armour, the huge American sportswear firm, is trying very hard to sign up Real Madrid to wear their kit. They are offering a massive €150 million a season to prise Real away from the clutches of Adidas.

After that, of course, they may have to deal with all the separate deals players have with various kit providers. Ronaldo might wear Under Armour on match days. Getting him to wear the gear in photos that accompany interviews or when he is being filmed is a different kettle of fish.

Meanwhile, Under Armour are trying to cover their own arses on the home front too. The biggest star in their growing galaxy is Steph Curry, the gifted leader of the Golden State Warriors NBA franchise. Recently he took exception to Under Armour's chairman Kevin Plank praising President Donald Trump for his pro-business stance: 'a real asset for this country', Plank said. Various UA-contracted players and celebs demurred. Curry said, 'I agree with that description if you remove the "et" from asset.'

The same week, Nike proved themselves to be a bit more in tune with the zeitgeist when they rolled out a multimedia advertising campaign based on 'equality'.

That is the world professional sports has become. There is a febrile connection between leading brands and leading stars and teams. Everybody loves each other and 'shares the same beliefs', until something goes wrong. Ask Tiger Woods or Lance Armstrong what happened to all the corporate love when things turned bad for them. On the other side of the equation, ask Kevin Plank.

Sponsors and brands are there to sell stuff. If players and clubs get rich helping, that is a happy coincidence. Only fools mistake the relationship for love.

You'll remember Petr Cech's head injury. When he eventually returned to football he had to wear a protective cap. Sportswear manufacturers Canterbury, being rugby people, obviously had a range of these, but Adidas flipped at the thought of him wearing something with the Canterbury logo on it. Within weeks they had provided him with spanking-new Adidas-branded head protection.

We walk in a minefield. You see that Lucozade bottle on the side of the pitch? More than likely it's not full of Lucozade. It's full of water, or the specific drink the club or player wants to use. Players have to be seen to be slugging from a Lucozade bottle though.

I remember a goalie who used to stash a can of Red Bull in his goal along with his towels and spare gloves. He got a letter from the Premier League telling him that Red Bull wasn't an official sponsor. He had to cease and desist. Should have decanted it into a Lucozade bottle.

We might use Evian water but we have to take all the labels

off the bottles before we go out. This week we are playing a last-sixteen game in the Champions League. The first leg is away from home. On the school run, parents ask me if I am excited. Of course I say yes. They imagine every trip I go on is like a city break, except with better-looking people and nicer hotels. It seems churlish to tell them that when we have Champions League games abroad or at home we have to spend a lot of time taking every label off every water bottle and piece of medical kit. No branded product can appear *anywhere* on a Champions League night.

I have an Umbro bag for my physio stuff. The little bag I run on to the field with. (Once every few years some wit on the team gets the idea to hide it. Like clockwork, I freak out. There is great amusement, and I have to explain that there are drugs in the bag and me 'losing' the bag is not really that funny for me.) All and any of the logos on things like my medical bag have to be covered up with tape. Technically I am supposed to use an official Champions League medical bag. They're crap, so I don't want to use an official Champions League bag. That's why I painstakingly tape over every logo on my Umbro bag.

Players' boots are another battlefield where design and style outweigh comfort and performance. Branding overrides everything though. With one player who wanted a spat-strapping – common in American football, where the tape goes over the boot – we found that it covered the identity of the bootmaker. Crisis. We had to draw the bootmaker's logo on top of the tape just to keep the sponsors happy.

So we're off to Europe again. We won't be seeing the sights or

245

sampling the local culture, but we will be working hard to keep one step ahead of the global branding police.

Leicester City are struggling. Last year's Premier League champions are dangling by a thread just above the relegation canyon. The media, always piercingly sharp in their analysis, have been interrogating Claudio Ranieri about pizza and pasta. No pizza this year then? Is it true that some of the players don't like the pre-game pasta meals?

Ranieri confused everybody by announcing that even as a gentleman who has always been openly Italian, he doesn't really like pasta. He added that the players have fried chicken before games.

What? Jamie Vardy's having a party . . . bucket?

Everything the media thought they knew is wrong, it seems.

The foreign influence on English football is a funny thing. It has developed slowly over the years. I have seen many managers from very different cultures. They vary. Some are hugely into the dietary side of things. Other managers are happy enough for a player to have a glass of wine at the table. Italian clubs might have a glass of Chianti served with the players' lunches. If that was introduced at an English club the interpretation would be different. In other countries a drop of wine may be appropriate but in England we are still endeavouring to outgrow the infamous 'drinking clubs' and ten-pints-of-lager-and-a-packet-of-crisps dietary regimes.

I am interested in the different dietary trends we have seen come and go. We have gone from the tyranny of plain pasta and boiled vegetables to an insistence on tasty, interesting, nutritious food and an emphasis on eating together as a team.

Leicester are still in the Champions League and the FA Cup. If they somehow turn their PL season around perhaps we'll all be chomping KFC next year.

This morning I'm thinking of all the players I have treated down the years who have been heroic warriors when a high ball has been delivered into a crowded penalty area. In the era of tiki-taka that element of the game has declined in some countries, but in England we still enjoy the spectacle of big centre-halves having aerial battles with flying centre-forwards. Meaty headers made by players who don't care where they stick their heads so long as it is in the direction of the ball.

It makes me shudder.

The management of head injuries in football has become a lot more stringent over the last few years. In the past, when I attended players on the field who had been knocked unconscious, if they had quickly recovered and had no obvious symptoms, they carried on playing. (If I recall correctly, The Secret Footballer was once spun 360 degrees, landed semi-conscious in a heap but carried on playing!) This would not happen now. The rules have changed and the medics entering the field have a greater understanding of the dangers of head injuries. They are particularly cautious these days because they can be scrutinized on a television replay.

A player doesn't have to be rendered unconscious to suffer a concussion. Symptoms vary from headaches, dizziness and nausea to memory loss, balance disturbances and even changes in behaviour. If a player shows any of these symptoms he comes off the pitch for further assessment. And you need to be careful: I remember asking one player what the score was in our last game and who the Prime Minister was and he had no idea – not because he had a head injury, he just didn't know. After that I learned to make the questions relevant to the player, e.g. What is the name of Peter Crouch's missus?

Following the head injury, the player is then closely monitored and follows a Graduated Return to Play protocol (GRTP) which involves progressive increases in activity, ensuring that symptoms do not recur. In larger clubs, where there is an enhanced care setting with an excellent team of clinicians monitoring this process, this can take as little as six days. For Under-19s the GRTP takes a minimum of twelve days, with complete rest being mandatory for the first seven days.

Multiple head injuries (or even head impact such as when heading the ball) can have a cumulative effect on a player. The Reading, Wolves and Republic of Ireland striker Kevin Doyle followed medical advice to retire from football at the age of thirty-four. He had made a total of 490 club and 75 international appearances, but towards the end of his career he increasingly suffered episodes of concussive symptoms, sometimes simply by heading a ball. More recently, Ryan Mason of Hull City, who clashed heads with Chelsea's Gary Cahill in January 2017 and sustained a fractured skull, was advised not to play again because his ongoing symptoms did not resolve themselves.

Chronic damage in the brain has been seen in 99 per cent of NFL players and is now more frequently occurring in footballers who played during the 1960s and 1970s. CTE (chronic traumatic encephalopathy) is a neurodegenerative disease found in those who have suffered multiple head injuries. The most notable case of CTE was the West Bromwich Albion and England international Jeff Astle, who went on to develop dementia; it was identified that his brain had marked changes indicative of CTE. Reports from families of footballers of the 1966 World Cup squad indicate that they are also now suffering from similar problems.

And just to bring things right up to date . . . the FA and PFA embarked on a study in early 2018 to look at the physical and mental health of about fifteen thousand former players and compare them to the wider population. This is the first study of its kind to try and identify the impact that playing football can have on the brain. We await the findings with keen interest, even if it leads to delaying heading of the ball in our younger, developing players.

Meanwhile, our job here in the medical room remains the same: to help and protect young players. In the years that I have been involved in football we have become enlightened enough that players don't have their long-term health jeopardized for the short-term gain of teams. We don't send players out with knees shot full of cortisone and we don't have crazy training sessions where players carry each other up and down terraces almost guaranteeing damage to their joints. We give them the best available information and try to restrict them to best practices.

I have known pain myself. When I left my previous job where I had been running the medical department for many years, I was surprised to hear some supporters bring up the fact that it was the medical team, particularly me, that was responsible for some of the long-term injuries.

Not only did it amaze me how good fans' memories are, it also surprised me how little they know about the causative factors of injury and injury management. They seemed strangely unwilling to sit down and listen to an introductory lecture on the subject. So here goes . . .

The causes of injury are either intrinsic (player specific) or extrinsic (external factors). Intrinsically, the main causes of injury are age and previous form: older players get injured more, and if you have had an injury previously, you are at a greater risk of re-injuring that same area again. The club can't do anything about either of these factors – apart from refraining from signing injury-prone old players in the first place.

Preventing injury is the Holy Grail of sports medicine. There are many theories on the subject, mostly unproven. These include strength training, stretching, yoga, Pilates, functional movement screening, balance exercises . . . I could go on and on. Indeed I often do. I can tell players all this, but when they are not at the club I have to rely on them to help themselves.

Essentially, injury prevention is specific to the player. A prevention strategy is different from one player to another as their needs are all different. There is, however, really only one influential factor that extrinsically causes players to get injured, and that is training load.

Training influences a player's fitness level and his ability to be 'football fit'. If they are not fit enough, they will break in games as their system has not been conditioned properly for match play. If training is excessive, they will break due to over-stressing the system.

The specific aspects of training have to be balanced and tai-lored. In training, you want to improve technique but not too much to cause fatigue and injury. A common issue is when the team practises crossing and shooting. In a match situation, crossing or shooting happens numerous times if you are a wide player or striker, but in training *all* players in *all* positions tend to be involved and as many as fifty crosses can be attempted in one session. But how often does a centre-half cross a ball in a game? This results in many players complaining of tight groins.

And when it comes to niggles and knocks, it is naive to think that, within a professional football club, it is the sole responsi-bility of the medical team to decide when a player is fit to return. At times, the manager, coaching staff, fitness coach, sports scientist, board members, the player himself, family (especially with the younger players) and even his agent can all get involved in the decision-making process.

It is about managing risk, and this has to be a team decision, even if we, the medical team, don't like it and the fans generally just don't want to know about it.

I mention all this because we have got to the end of February, out of the FA Cup but still alive in the Champions League and in third place contending for the title, with injury rates negli-gible. The games are going to be coming thick and fast. Good. Having games twice a week at the back end of the season is a benefit as far as I can see.

Firstly, that's how it's supposed to be. Success leads to more games. And playing constantly cements the conditioning of players and frees them from the perils of being given the odd excessive training session as reprisal for a loss. Two or even three games per week do bring with them an increased risk of injury, but you have to reduce training accordingly. Monitoring with GPS during training and matches helps the sports scientists to minimize this risk.

Basically, all the team will be doing for the next couple of months is playing and resting. And when you're in a rhythm, everybody is happy. (Unless, as José Mourinho points out, you are in the Europa League and might end up playing seventy games in a season as punishment for not making the Champions League.)

Elsewhere, poor Claudio Ranieri got whacked a couple of weeks after his board promised they would never allow such a thing to happen. Then his former players, widely accused of treachery themselves, went out and beat Liverpool while under the guidance of a caretaker manager. Liverpool have lost five in seven, so now Jürgen Klopp of Liverpool (and La Manga) is looking over his shoulder. He signed something like a thousand-year contract early in his time at Anfield. That doesn't mean a man can't get whacked though.

Thank heavens I am but a humble physio. Sometimes this job is pretty good, even if nobody ever chants a physio's name from the terrace!

TSF: Second Opinion

Heads up

Thankfully, footballers are listening to their bodies now far more than they ever used to. Perhaps we've always been guilty of masking the odd knock, but given that players are becoming quicker, more athletic and stronger, a knock to the head isn't something that we can just run off any more or, worse, ignore.

And I have been as guilty as any player when it comes to ignoring medical advice and carrying on after a concussion. It was coming towards the end of another Premier League season and it was well known that Aston Villa were in the market that summer for a player in my position with the same traits that I specialized in. I had the words of my agent ringing in my ears: 'If you have just one good game this season make sure it's this one.' Martin O'Neill had already made it clear that the club would bid for me that summer and all I needed to do was get through the game at Villa Park with my body and my reputation intact.

Fifteen minutes into the game I was knocked out cold after a clash of heads with a Villa player. I'd actually made a good start but I knew that my work for this weekend at least was all but over. Except that it wasn't.

In such situations it is customary for a player to run through the motions with his physio. Like a boxer on a standing count, he sways in a wind that doesn't exist while telling whoever his eyes focus on that he's OK to carry on.

I was not OK and yet I was allowed to play on. It was a huge mistake all round. I've since watched the video back and I can see my legs bowing as the physio helps me up. I'm all over the place. I've since wondered why it is that referees do not make it their business to assess players on the pitch; if they are unsure of a player's ability to continue they should be able to ask for the opinion of an independent doctor at pitchside. Clubs always have their own doctor present in any case, but in the interests of fair play an independent doctor might be a better bet.

I was put out of my misery on the hour mark after a string of passes that were blighted by blurred vision and decision-making that would have made a Tory front bench look competent. Martin O'Neill didn't call my agent back.

I should have come off for the sake of my body and my reputation, but football does strange things to players even when their heads are seemingly clear. The concern is that football will do even stranger things to players long after they've retired.

Fat club

The dreaded fat club. The cause of early-morning misery to so many footballers who subscribe to the theory that fatness is like a virus. You catch it and it is the club's responsibility to deal with it, especially in pre-season. It's a virus you catch in Las Vegas around the pool after twenty chilled Coronas but a virus nonetheless. An act of God.

Fat club is where you go if you are fatter when you came back from your pre- or mid-season trip than you were when the physio last measured your body mass index. Cure? Get up at eight a.m., get to training before anybody else and start running around that training pitch, you big fat cunt!

Football is behind the curve when it comes to body shaming.

I can afford to be scathing. Not because I look after myself overly well, but because God or whoever my manufacturer was knew that I was a lazy bastard and took the precaution of making sure that I would not suffer from telltale deposits of porky stuff around my midriff. No matter what I eat or drink, or in what quantity, I stay thin.

That is my superpower. Or, as my wife calls it, my one redeeming feature.

You thought the anonymity was a branding thing? Nah. Policing the crowds of women who wanted a piece of a fat-proof footballer just took too many men off the streets. I put society's needs ahead of my own.

Generally, for those who haven't been genetically fat-proofed there is no excuse or sympathy. Yes, the lower down you go in professional football you'll find more players who are life members of the fat club, but I've seen players at Premier League level who could serve as poster boys for the club if the posters were landscape-shaped and not portrait.

Being a sin that I find it hard to commit, I thus find it unforgivable. I have no sympathy.

And if you're going to spray your Instagram account with images of you drinking champagne from the bottle while surrounded by the great and the riddled of the global nightlife scene, then you get what you fucking deserve when you come back.

You know who you are!

Fuckbit

I once played at a club where the physio was either progressive or a little bit creepy. It really depends on your liberalism. He'd manage to turn most rehabilitation techniques into their sexual counterpart.

When I strained my rectus femoris muscle – at the top of the thigh – he said, 'You have to encourage the fibres to knit back together by gently stressing the leg backwards and forwards.' As you know, when you stress muscle fibre it breaks up but heals far stronger than when you started. It's the same principle as bodybuilders lifting weights.

He would say to me, 'What you really need is to have sex with your missus doggy style, and just gently flex the rec fem for fifteen minutes backwards and forwards. That's the perfect treatment for this.'

He also used to say to the manager that the lads who were in the fat club should just have more sex with their partners. 'Fifteen hundred calories on average,' he'd say, 'in fifteen minutes.' To my mind that beats plodding endlessly around a training pitch in the baking heat of summer.

Years later, when Fitbits came out, my wife borrowed one from a friend and we tested the theory. It really works: fifteen minutes burns 1,500 calories, folks. Why the fuck would you ever go for a run again?

Dodgy Rodge

There is a man in Leicester called Oldham who should really be part of a limerick.

> There's a doctor in Leicester called Oldham
> Who'll sugar your ligaments and remould 'em.
> For a little wonga
> He'll make you much stronger –
> Sadly not much rhymes with Oldham, I told him.

So, as he's called Dr Roger Oldham, and we footballers are in too much of a hurry to think of anything better, we call him Dodgy Rodge because Dodge, as you may have copped, rhymes with Rodge.

Which is pretty harsh on a great professional who is available day or night and who has the ability to save a player's career with nothing more than a jab into a ligament of sugar syrup mixed with phenol and glycerol. Dr Oldham's prolotherapy is actually the only miracle cure I've seen since my mother told my brother that if he didn't get up from his bed of death and go to school he'd have to spend the day tidying his room.

Dr Rodge has saved my career on at least three occasions.

You don't have to have had medical training to know that the news about your ligament is bad when they scan you. A damaged ligament will reveal itself as a black void on an ultrasound scan. A healthy ligament will reveal itself as a beautiful solid white fibrous mass. The first time I visited Dr Oldham my knee looked like a black hole. One that had been swallowed by another much larger black hole.

Nothing had worked.

Prolotherapy was to be my saviour. The fluid is injected straight into the ligament and hardens what is already there immediately. That encourages new tissue to grow. It's simple and fucking effective and it's drug-free. Dr Oldham doesn't even use radiography to map out the territory; he goes by feel and touch. The injections inflame the ligaments in a controlled way and promote healing. If you want to see Dr Rodge in action just google the words 'Andrew Morris and prolotherapy'. The transatlantic rower had just about given up on his back ever feeling good again, but . . .

In the US prolotherapy is common practice, particularly in the NFL where knee and ankle ligament injuries are common, and because of the very lateral lines players take in the course of a game the odd jab here and there is perfect. But in the UK, when I played at least, Dr Rodge was pretty much the only doctor practising this treatment in the country.

Over the years I saw Dr Rodge for every ligament injury I ever had. I saw him when one particular Premier League player, who shall remain nameless (like myself, to be fair), tried to end my career by destroying my knee. He has since come to a bad end (career-wise) himself but I still have no feeling in my knee after a tackle that left me with nerve damage. When the nerves are kaput it's almost impossible to tell whether or not you are healed and fit to play again. No sense of pain, no sense of gain.

My wife used to sit in on the treatment sessions. I thought at the time that she came along for the excellent tuna sandwiches which got served up after a session. Now I think she just enjoyed seeing me being punctured with large needles.

When you're having a jab at the local GP's the doctor says, 'OK, sharp scratch coming up . . . and here we go. That wasn't so bad, was it?' If Dr Roger had said, 'OK, alligator bite coming up, ready?' he wouldn't have been selling the experience short.

A needle required to reach the cruciate ligament is so long that it could be used for pole-vaulting. The pain involved in welcoming the needle into your ligament area is excruciating even if they inject you with a local anaesthetic before the main jab.

I've mentioned elsewhere the lengths we would go to just to relax me before the main jab. By lengths I mean pubs, and then Rohypnol. I would have married Dr Rodge, and whatever it took I would have borne him many children, if he had just given me a general anaesthetic. He used Rohypnol instead because he needed the body to respond naturally when he flexed my knee to make sure he'd put enough fluid in. If you go under a general your body becomes as limp as a rag doll and nobody can tell what the knee's natural response is.

Several times I wandered out of that Bupa hospital with an IV still in my arm and drove home while the hospital frantically tried to find out where I was. I remember bleeding all over the sofa at home once. I don't remember how I got home that day, only Mrs TSF pulling a little needle out of my arm and asking me what it was. I think it was after that that she began accompanying me.

Over time, Dr Rodge refined the technique and began to study the root cause of injury, particularly soft-tissue injuries like hamstrings, groin strains and back complaints. What he has discovered is to my mind brilliant and totally underused in this country.

During one trip he said to me, 'I bet you have a weak right ankle, let me check.'

He flexed the ankle joint up and down.

Then the left ankle.

The right ankle was considerably more lax than the left.

'I don't know why this is the case but I find this same result in around 75 per cent of people. When I inject the ankle to stiffen it, the soft-tissue injuries dry up. I've got the whole of the Leicester Tigers squad coming in next week and to my mind every squad should have this done before every season.'

Now then, I am a cynical fucker and proud of it. It would make me genuinely sick if I turned out to be a sucker for the old placebo ruse. I swear, though, that the injection into my right ankle curtailed my soft-tissue injuries. I had a great season. I felt solid and strong all over. I implored my team-mates to have it done but footballers are creatures of habit rather than desperation. The club would have kicked up a stink too. The jabs are £1,000 each.

But if I were a manager of a Premier League club I'd insist on it. I know it works.

So cheers for saving my career, Dr Rodge, and for the right ankle that will forever point towards Leicester.

MARCH

At matches, as in life, I'm always one step behind everybody else.

At key moments I'm looking at where the ball has been to make sure that our player has got up and I'm checking there's no reaction if there has been a tackle. I'm watching for a player who either doesn't get up or who gets up limping. I try to keep in communication with both the tunnel doc and the team doc sitting next to me. Often one of us will watch the player while the other watches the game. But there is always some cocky coach who will ask me if I've not noticed some player struggling on the pitch. I'm not stupid. I know he's been struggling for a few minutes.

Last night, when we scored a late winner ten minutes from time, we went joint top of the Premier League. OK we have played an extra game, but it was a huge moment.

I wasn't aware of which player had scored or how he had done it till about an hour after the game. In the build-up, our attacking midfielder played one of those killer 15-yard passes along the grass taking out two defenders. For his trouble he got taken out late. I was already grabbing my bag when I heard the crowd roar and saw the other players streak past the fallen colleague on their way to celebrate.

In the stadium there was bedlam, but I had voices in both my ears. The coaches were celebrating and hugging and had hardly noticed the injury. The referee and linesman were getting ready to restart the match. I was on the touchline like the fool on the hill, standing perfectly still. Waiting. In my ear, after what seemed like an age, the physio in the changing room was describing the injury as he was seeing it on slow-motion replay after the live feed had stopped showing the goal.

At games we try to have one of the medical team watching the game from a medical room down the tunnel. He seldom sees daylight, and informs the medical staff of each team about what he has seen on the replays of injuries.

Now the curious thing is that, as everybody over the age of ten knows, the technology is there to let us view replays of injuries ourselves at pitchside. We can sit where we normally sit with tablets or portable devices and watch any replay when we need to, just as they do in rugby. That would be the common-sense approach. I have read that the reason for not having replays available on the bench is that it would be a performance advantage (but surely not if both teams had the same technology?). So we aren't allowed to do that. Apparently officials aren't permitted to view replays during a match – there are no screens in the dugout any more. Instead, we use our guy in the back room. It is he who studies the footage to ascertain the mechanism of an injury and then transmits these details to me or the opposition medical staff via radio. What we should have is full access to as much information as possible, as quickly as possible.

(But be careful what you wish for . . . the introduction during the 2017-18 season of the video assistant referee (VAR) has certainly been controversial. Important decisions have been taking an age to resolve, and in some cases the tempo of the game has been directly affected. After an FA Cup fourth-round tie with Liverpool at the end of January, West Brom manager Alan Pardew branded the technology a 'farce' after two of his players pulled hamstrings when their muscles contracted in the cold weather during the lengthy delays. That's bad enough, but there is also a feeling that VAR isn't providing us with anything like the quality of information most had expected, that rather than giving us black and white answers it's simply continuing to muddy a grey palette. West Brom had a goal disallowed following a VAR referral even though most pundits and fans who watched the same replay agreed Craig Dawson's effort should have stood. Clearly there is more work to be done, and anybody who works in the game should be a sucker for more information, but we must ask ourselves to what lengths we're prepared to go in order to get it.)

Certainly once I'm on the field and treating a player it can be useful to have the replays replayed and commentated upon in my ear: our man may have seen the incident two or three times by the time I get to the player. He can tell me if the player has lost consciousness and/or where the impact was. By the time I am coming on the player may be coming to. I need to know what happened to him. Often, though, the best thing is for me actually to see the mechanics of the injury for myself.

Behind the scenes there is also the tunnel doctor, a very useful innovation. It's the tunnel doc who liaises with the away-team doctor, informing the visitors about the facilities and later providing support for any injuries or emergencies. The presence of a tunnel doctor is increasingly important in an era when we have become more conscious of the proper protocol for head injuries. A player who comes off with a knock to the head is now continuously assessed and monitored for deterioration of clinical symptoms. If a player is taken to hospital during the match, the tunnel doc remains at the home stadium ensuring that two doctors are still present.

If the player has lost consciousness then he has to come off, which often doesn't go down well with him or his manager. If he's not pulled off the field the club will get caned on the television, and in turn I'll get caned later on. I can't always tell from afar whether or not the player has been knocked out – he might have been, briefly, but come to by the time I get to him. He might tell me that he's OK but the television cameras will show what really happened.

There is also other less vital information that regularly comes through my earpiece, such as, 'Hey mate, look, there's a really cute steward to your left.' Or, as they know we have our backstage medic on the radio, the coaches may be asking me 'Was that a free kick?' or 'Was that a handball?'

I have to answer.

'Yeah, it was a foul.'

'Aw fucking hell.'

And the coach runs straight over to the fourth official.

The official is taken aback and he's asking, 'Well how would you know? How do you know that?'

'Look, I just know.'

Sometimes you go on the pitch and as soon as you arrive the coach with the radio is in your ear like a fretting mother.

'Is he all right? Is he OK? Is he coming off?'

'Give me a minute, mate. I can't tell just by looking in his direction as I run across.'

And some days it's all so noisy that I can't hear what anyone is saying anyway.

Suits me. Being able to review the injury myself, without all the distraction – that would suit me even better.

Three of the academy kids got released today. It happens all the time but you can't help but feel for them. Two were ear-marked as goners a while back, but the other lad had really looked as if he was going to make it. He was tough and skilful and seemed like he wanted it badly. He was also a little bit mad in the head. At a youth tournament last summer he got caught red-handed inhaling nitrous oxide. It wasn't his first disciplinary offence. He was a good kid at heart I believe, but too immature to get it into his head that laughing gas is no laughing matter.

Over the past few months there has been an increasing number of players inhaling recreational drugs of some kind or another. For a while now we have been used to reading the stories about Arsenal and England midfielder Jack Wilshere getting caught on social media when out drinking booze, or smoking cigarettes or shisha pipes. This sort of thing has been going on for years and footballers are just a reflection of youth experimenting with new things. Their mates are doing it, they feel, so why shouldn't they?

But the increase in the use of nitrous oxide (NO), or 'laughing gas', or 'hippy crack', is perhaps the most concerning of the lot. In recent times, Liverpool's Raheem Sterling, Stoke's new striker Saido Berahino and Jack Grealish of Aston Villa have all been caught using the popular drug.

In 2013-14, apparently, over 470,000 people between the ages of sixteen and fifty-nine used NO, which was an increase of 100,000 on the previous year. It is – and this surprised me – the second most commonly used recreational drug behind cannabis. Cannabis can be picked up in dope tests but NO cannot. It is cheap, too, at about £2 a hit, and legal to buy if you are over eighteen. So for a young player it seems like a win-win. Until somebody catches you red-handed.

So what is nitrous oxide? NO is the canister gas used to make whipped cream frothy and light. That's not what you wanted to know though, is it? It's also the gas we medics use to kill pain when a player sustains a severe injury such as a broken leg. Commonly known as Entonox. You might have had some at the dentist's. You take a few deep breaths and the pain you were feeling significantly lessens. Other effects of inhaling the gas include a dizzy high lasting for about one minute, and some confusion and hallucinations. So you can see the attraction.

Feelings of numbness and tingling are common, but it is stressed (does NO come with serving suggestions?) that if these are felt, the user should stop immediately to avoid further serious effects occurring. Of course by then the user may feel drunk and incurably giggly.

In the wrong hands, therefore, it can even be deadly. A report in 2012 attributed fifty-two deaths over a thirty-year period to the use of NO. This was usually as a result of asphyxiation as the gas was inhaled in an enclosed area. That's not a catastrophic figure, but recreational use of the gas has increased massively since that study was taken.

Other dangers include collapse and subsequent injury, especially when mixed with alcohol. This is the worry that clubs have about their valuable players. In addition, regular use of NO inactivates the vitamin B12, which can lead to effects such as nerve damage due to vitamin deficiency. All in all that's a fairly hefty bill for a very short buzz.

So the club let a good young player go today, partly because he made a stupid mistake and partly because they needed to demonstrate to others that this particular error has grave consequences. I'm fairly certain that the survivors in the academy won't follow in the footsteps of their departed mate.

The word around the club today was that the kid has joined a pretty grim non-league club for the rest of the season.

We all got to say those words again: no laughing matter. Ha ha.

Hopefully the career of the departed player will recover, but I am doubtful. Meanwhile, I will have to keep a closer eye on my trusty medical bag to make sure it doesn't end up in one of the players' cars.

We are at home tonight in the second leg of our Champions League tie and barring disaster there will be more big nights like this to look forward to in the coming weeks. The Champions League is an end in itself and it gets more exciting the deeper into the competition you get. Even if we get knocked out at this stage we have something to be thankful for.

We aren't in the Europa League. Hallelujah! The Europa League doesn't really cut it in terms of excitement or prestige – ask anyone. Clubs see it as an inferior competition to the Champions League, almost like a cruel reprimand for last season's failure, a measly consolation prize. You didn't make the top four, and if you are a club where a top four placing is expected and demanded, the Europa League is what happens to you. If you are celebrating getting into the Europa League the chances are that your squad isn't big enough for anything more, or you're just happy for the rarity of European football. I think the year Chelsea won the thing they played just short of seventy games all told. Shudder.

If your league placing doesn't put you in the Europa League, then your group campaign in the Champions League going badly will, and then you have the ignominy of being shunted into the last 480 (or whatever it is) of the competition and you get to play matches in places you have never heard of on Thursday nights (which messes up the weekly timetables). The travelling is the worst. Even destinations that might be interesting to explore don't sound too appetizing from a football point of view.

Even the name doesn't help . . . Europa sounds *soooo* Euro-trashy. I much prefer the 'UEFA Cup'. It's the same trophy so I don't understand why they changed the name. Probably spent a few million on a marketing consultancy for that one.

So whatever happens tonight, we have dodged the bullet that is the Europa League.

A top football club is run on the same principles as a top stable for thoroughbreds. Except that players get to wander out of the paddock and into the big bad dangerous real world most afternoons.

While they are at the club, though, they are looked after in every way so that their lives are geared towards football and the business of being better footballers. As a reward for this they are given an obscene amount of oats.

They are literally tended to from toe to head. Most clubs provide access to experts, from chiropodists and podiatrists to shrinks with all stops in between also catered for. Sunderland used to have a hairdressing salon at the training ground!

Of all the services available, the one the players seem to dread most is the dentist. (It's also the kind of care most players, even at the highest level, will fund themselves, under the club medics' referral.) The dentist is very necessary though, not only when there is an acute issue where a player's tooth is chipped or knocked out but in terms of general oral hygiene.

Here is something the tabloids won't tell you girls (or guys): you should think twice before kissing a footballer.

A recent study (2015) published in the *British Journal of Sports Medicine* revealed the shockingly grotty dental state of some of our Premier League and Football League players. A total of 187 players, from clubs including Manchester United, Southampton, Swansea City, West Ham United, Hull City, Brighton & Hove Albion, Cardiff City and Sheffield United, were examined by dentists from the International Centre for Evidence-Based Oral Health. Their findings sent shockwaves through the world of WAGs and concerned mothers. More than four out of ten players had tooth decay (in the population at large, it affects one in three). Seventy-seven per cent had at least one filling, with the average number being five. Seventy-seven per cent had gingivitis affecting over half of their mouths and 5 per cent had moderate to severe irreversible gum/jaw disease.

Remember Alan Mullery damaging his back while brushing his teeth? Apparently a lot of players are declining to take that risk.

Forty-five per cent were 'actively bothered' by their oral health and one-fifth of players said that it reduced their overall quality of life. It affected what they ate because they suffered from intense sensitivity, and gave them problems at night. And you always thought that 'problems at night' for a player meant paparazzi outside a nightclub.

The study also revealed that 7 per cent of players said the state of their gnashers had affected their training or perform-ance. And this has been backed up by many other studies linking poor dental health with injury. The results varied from club to club, some having few problems and others a lot more.

Clubs such as West Ham have had major problems with play-ers in the past, which has resulted in improvements in oral hygiene management and education. In 2012, Ravel Morrison was sent home from a pre-season tour to have seven teeth removed. The bill came to more than £28,000 and he missed a significant part of the important pre-season preparation period.

He's never been quite the same since.

He isn't the only well-known player to have bad railings. Remember the gappy, protruding teeth of Ronaldo, Ronaldinho and Luis Suárez? (But good for biting, eh Luis?) And the gorgeous smile, merely lacking four front teeth, of Leeds United striker Joe Jordan? And let's not forget Carlos Tevez, whose teeth were damaged after a street fight when he was growing up in the violent town of Fuerte Apache (with a name like that he should have known), near Buenos Aires in Argentina. But all these examples were a result of trauma or bad genes, not poor dental health and hygiene.

This problem affects other athletes, too. The football study's author, Professor Ian Needleman of University College London, previously did a study of 2012 Olympians and found that these athletes' teeth were in a similar state, or even worse. Athletes have problems due to a lot of air in the mouth during exercise, which dries out the interior resulting in less 'protective saliva'.

Another suggested reason for the high incidence of oral problems in sport is the use of sugary drinks. Yet although two-thirds of footballers consumed a sugary drink at least three times a week, this was not found to be significant and no correlation between such beverages and tooth decay was found.

At our club, the use of isotonic drinks has declined over the past few years, with fewer players drinking them for fluid replacement. Many prefer to use plain water, or add calorie-free flavouring tablets to water to improve palatability. Some opt to use milk-based drinks that have been shown to rehydrate athletes quicker than water. We advise our players to swish their mouths out with water after drinking a sugary fluid – an attempt to 'wash some of it away' to prevent the sugar sitting on the teeth.

But if sugary drinks aren't the main cause, what is? One idea is that many players grow up in impoverished communities or developing countries where there is poor dental care and education. This may lead to problems with teeth from an early age. Even something as simple as being taught how to clean your teeth properly – doing so before eating food, or twenty minutes after, to allow the saliva to cleanse and protect the teeth – is a fundamental life habit. They say you're supposed to supervise your kids until they are twelve or something. Blimey, I haven't got time for that.

Ideally, this comes from parents. But this is where academies are useful too, as frequently it's the parents who need educating. At our club, a dental examination is part of the pre-signing medical. Even with his mesmerizing stepovers and nifty rabona, Shane MacGowan never really had a chance in the beautiful game.

The level of medical care at professional football games has come a long way over the past twenty years.

When I first started in football, I remember players whose warm-up consisted of standing in a hot bath, and instead of a Red Bull for a caffeine pick-me-up they would have a swig from the physio's 'magic' bottle. Only their expression afterwards would indicate how strong what was inside must have been. Back then, many a drugs test would have been failed. I heard that the legendary West Ham physio Rob Jenkins occasionally gave players a swig of a potent alcoholic 'livener'.

As happens so often in life, it takes a major incident for people to take notice of a problem or shortcoming and embark upon change. In the field of football medicine internationally, this occurred after the on-field death of Marc-Vivien Foé in 2003, Petr Cech suffering a fractured skull three years later in the UK and the near-death incident in March 2012 involving Fabrice Muamba.

How they were managed, both during and afterwards, was terrible, and each has since been closely scrutinized to learn what went wrong. The image of Foé's open, fixed eyes and limp arm hanging as he was stretchered off the pitch, with no one administering any type of life support or care, was truly haunting. The only saving grace in the case of the Cech incident was that, despite the inferior care provided, he returned to full competitive play. Since that October day in 2006 when Reading played Chelsea in a foul-tempered game and Cech suffered that freakish injury, so much in the game has changed for us medics.

After Cech, that change came in terms of how to manage a head injury. Now we would immobilize the player following such an incident. That day people were sitting Cech up to see if he could carry on. He was stretchered off and left unattended in the changing room (well, with a masseur or some such, not with somebody who could resuscitate him if he bled internally and collapsed). He should have been spinal-boarded, collared and taken straight to hospital. His life was in the balance right until he had metal plates successfully inserted in his head at the John Radcliffe Hospital in Oxford.

Weirdly, in the same game Ibrahima Sonko of Reading wiped out Carlo Cudicini, the substitute goalkeeper. John Terry had to go in goal. Both Chelsea keepers ended up in hospital in the same match.

When Dean Kenneally, the then Chelsea physio, and Bryan English, the doctor, reached Petr Cech that day there weren't many clues as to the danger the keeper was in. Cech was conscious and was speaking to his doctor. Good signs normally. He managed to crawl off the field of play. When he was eventually stretchered off down the tunnel to the dressing room he was still conversing, but after a few minutes English could see that the keeper was in more trouble than had at first seemed to be the case. He asked for an ambulance.

English had to return to the pitch for another injury in what was a fiery game. When he came back in, the situation had deteriorated. He asked again about the ambulance.

Cech was first brought to the local Royal Berkshire Hospital before being transferred to Oxford hours later after a scan highlighted the precise danger. The early collision with the leg of Reading midfielder Stephen Hunt had dented Cech's fragile skull. Pieces of bone had been pushed towards the brain.

And still we learned at a snail's pace. It's only a few years since we had the disturbing incident of the then Spurs manager André Villas-Boas insisting on sending his goalkeeper Hugo Lloris back on to the field of play after a transient episode of unconsciousness. By the time the Spurs doctor and physio had reached him, Lloris was conscious again. The medics then had to assess his ability to carry on. They wanted him to come off. Their manager overrode the decision.

It could be that communication was poor and the gravity of the situation was not adequately emphasized to AVB. But it was worrying to see the manager so defiant after the incident. 'The call always belongs to me,' Villas-Boas said. He had been one of Chelsea's coaching staff at the time of the Petr Cech incident so of all people he should have been erring on the side of caution.

A similar incident happened to the Uruguayan Álvaro Pereira and the German international Christoph Kramer during the 2014 World Cup. Both were allowed to play on, although the Uruguay doc tried his best to stop Pereira from doing so.

Fabrice Muamba sparked another set of medical protocol changes six years after Cech's injury following his on-field cardiac arrest while playing for Bolton against Spurs. The memory of distressed players crying as medics performed CPR on Muamba is again something that haunts football. After seven long minutes he was stretchered into an ambulance where a heart specialist who just happened to be in the crowd that day was waiting, having stepped forward.

Before these three incidents happened, I had no formal training to manage heart attacks, head injuries or concussion. My management was based on logic rather than learned skills and many times I got away with it. Today in the UK we have compulsory FA-run courses relating to head injuries for medical staff, with top-ups annually. If you don't pass the exams you're not allowed to go on the pitch. Period. Whether or not an injured player stays on the field is the team doctor's decision, and no one else can override it. We are learning that when it comes to serious incidents such as head injuries and cardiac problems all decision-making needs to be removed from managers.

Staff working for Premier League and Championship clubs now attend many courses, but I have concerns about the lower divisions and non-league football. For me, basic life support and resuscitation should not only be a fundamental skill taught to all medics at games but all coaches too as part of their coaching badges. And even primary-school children. A five-year-old could competently use a defibrillator. It's a life skill. Why are we waiting for more tragedies to happen before we increase the chances of somebody present being in a position to do something to save a life? Is it because exposure and skill make us subconsciously put a different price on the life of a Premier League player than we put on a Sunday league footballer?

We gallop on into the final straight. It's getting hectic, but at this time of year if things are going well everyone at the club feels as if they are working together like parts of a machine. You have to keep going because if you don't the machine will break down.

We depend on each other, leaning on the expertise and experience of colleagues as we hurtle together through matches just keeping hope alive. It's a hard thing to express in words but it is a big part of what keeps me in football and makes all the annoying stuff worth enduring.

TSF: Second Opinion

If all else fails, try bribery

Your idea of bribery and corruption probably involves brown envelopes or expensive wristwatches being passed to FIFA execs in order to sway big decisions, or wads of cash passing through the hands of conniving agents to sweeten mega transfer deals.

How quaint.

Football has evolved. Bribery is now done by paying companies who are registered in that unknowable place we call offshore. The companies then clean the money and send it back. Nobody gets their hands dirty any more.

You will be glad to know, however, that more traditional forms of the corruption craft can still be found at local level.

The scourge of almost every professional footballer is the requirement to play in reserve games. Nobody likes it, nobody wants to do it. Traipsing to John O'Groats on a Tuesday night to play in a glorified youth team in front of one man and his reluctant dog is not living the dream.

When you bump into your senior colleagues on the opposite side, it is hard not to feel a little sheepish and embarrassed that you are both there. It's like running into a friend at an AA meeting. It goes without saying that you will keep it between yourselves.

We envy those senior pros who are coming back from long-term injuries. The first team has missed them and needs them. Some game time is a must. They aren't really slumming it like the rest of us. Reserve football is fine if you are injured and 'just passing through'. The humiliation comes when you just can't get a look-in with the first team.

Once, during a reserve match against Fulham, Paul Konchesky said to me, 'Mate, what the fuck are me and you doing here?'

I told him that I didn't know why I was there but I knew exactly why he was.

277

Never lose face, chaps.

Sometimes you get a manager who will insist on making you play in the reserves even if you have just had a knock that's kept you out for a week or two. This is a halfway house between humiliation and healing and is best avoided. It's as if the manager is saying to the physio, 'Look, I know he's OK to play, but the nineteen-year-old who has taken his place is doing well and the fans like him and he's only on 12K a week. Do we really need TSF? Really?'

This is when the physio can help you, and why I always befriended the physios in the way that Francis of Assisi cosied up to little birds. Having a little bird eating out of your hand is picture-postcard cute. Having a physio eating out of your hand is practical genius.

A nice physio gives you weekends off when you are injured and the team is playing away. A bad, horrible physio makes you come in to do some rehab work with a spotty lackey on work placement.

One has to play the game. Work hard during the week. If you don't work hard and do the rehab the physio's professionalism will beat your bribe every day of the week.

What you are paying for is the physio's ability to go to the manager and tell him categorically that putting the player back into training is far more beneficial than sending him 200 miles away to play against the Cardiff reserves.

It doesn't always have to be cash. In fact, cash seems vulgar. You can donate tickets, you remember to get boots for his son, you book a table for him and his lovely wife at a restaurant where your name has some clout. Honestly, the list is endless. It's all about using your imagination and finding his weaknesses.

It's old-fashioned, a craft and a tradition. It's wooing in the age of Tinder.

Physios get injured too

There is a club in English football called Middlesbrough. Honest. It's so far north you may not have heard of it. One trophy, I think. Can't remember what it was, but it is the sole major achievement of a club that was formed over a hundred years ago. That and losing in the final of the UEFA Cup to Seville. I'm told that in Middlesbrough they still close the streets every year when the anniversary of that particular achievement comes round.

Time was when Middlesbrough had a half-decent team; that is to say it was littered with players who would never have dared venture to Middlesbrough for any other reason than that there was a phenomenally bulbous cheque waiting for them when they stepped off the boat.

But even big players are capable of getting big injuries, and a few years ago one of Boro's biggest players had one of their biggest injuries.

Lots of physios try all sorts of different techniques to get their players fit again. For a midfielder, manoeuvrability is the key. He has to be able to move forward, back, left, right, up and down, like most players, but in the space of five yards, and it's tough. Really tough.

The midfielder was told by Boro's physio to play tennis with him. No game is better for a damaged soft-tissue injury than tennis. After all, the movement of a tennis player embodies all the traits of a Premier League midfielder.

After a set the midfielder was leading. But after three sets he was 2-1 down and fatigue, thanks to his time away from the pitch, was beginning to show. Frustration and competitiveness are a bad mix when a professional athlete can't do what his brain wants his body to do.

In the fourth set his stamina deserted him and the physio inflicted a mentally bruising defeat. The legendary midfielder wasn't going to take it lying down. With the last of his energy, he launched his tennis racket in the direction of his tormentor, only to see it split the physio's head open with alarming ease.

Fearing a fine in the tens of thousands of pounds, the midfielder rushed to the physio's aid and begged him to hush it up. Pride got the better of the physio who told the midfielder not to fret.

Alas, his pleas fell on deaf ears. Luckily for him. For the next day the midfielder issued an apology through the medium of bribery. A brand-new Rolex watch. Twenty grands' worth.

The midfielder? Well that'd be telling. Think short, black and Dutch.

And you thought being a physio was a shitty job.

Sleeping Beauty

As you all know by now, I suffer from depression. As a result I have a carefully tailored medicine cabinet that once allowed me to function as a human being and play professional football for a bunch of fucking massive clubs that didn't give a shit about my wellbeing so long as I did the business on the pitch. And more often than not, I did.

Of course, just like property, cars, watches, houses, girls, pensions and anything else, if one player looks as if he knows what he's doing in the changing room then he must know something that everybody wishes they knew.

Once upon a time I was that player. If I had a business plan everybody wanted to see it. If I had bought a new villa in Spain, everybody else wanted to know exactly where. If I had drugs, they wanted them.

Let me explain.

I had antidepressants. But I also had sleeping pills. And not just sleeping pills that send a standard-sized human being to sleep, but sleeping pills that could anaesthetize an entire herd of Indian elephants. Of course, my team-mates didn't know that.

So when a central defender came and knocked on my door one night before an away game, I was only too happy to hand over one of my tranquillizers.

The following day the central defender didn't materialize for breakfast. Nor for pre-match, nor for the video of the opposition. Finally one of the youth team had to get a key card to his room from reception and wake him up. We boarded the bus at 1.15 p.m. and drove to the stadium. Our central defender was fast asleep.

What followed has become the stuff of legend in football because the video footage still exists.

Our central defender was still sparko when the bus rocked up at the stadium. Unsurprisingly the defender was dropped for one of the youth-team players. I don't think he batted an eyelid.

The game began and we roared into a shitty 1-0 lead with half an hour left. We also hit the crossbar, but so what? Our manager was looking to shut up shop and so were a few of the players who were casting a few 'Any chance, gaffer?' glances over towards the touchline. The gaffer turned to look at his bench.

It is that image that has gone down in folklore.

The first sub was the goalkeeper. No. Not needed.

The second sub was a young black striker with pace to burn. The total opposite of what we needed at that moment.

The third sub was an ageing winger pretending that he could not give a shit what was happening. Definitely not.

The fourth sub was a young midfielder, a very generic player – he can play, but nobody is really sure where to play him or when to play him. Not the player we need in the midst of this battle.

The fifth sub is the man we need. An experienced centre-half who has been there and done it at the highest level. Perfect to see out the last twenty minutes in place of our ageing striker. He can rally the older pros around him and refocus the young players in the back line with him who are becoming mentally fatigued.

One problem: he's fast asleep against the side of the dugout. And I mean *fast* asleep. A Ryan Giggs solo run from his own goal line would not wake him.

Alas, we won the game by sending on the whippet and stringing six players across the middle of the pitch. We should have lost because the opposition had two glorious chances but thanks to the fact that some players are utterly shit, we survived.

God bless those tranquillizers.

Away days

We all have that one mate, don't we? Trigger. The guy who should keep his mouth shut but you're glad he didn't because you were going to ask the same question.

Sleeping pills sound like a common ancillary to healthcare. Like paracetamol. But sleeping pills border on the event horizon of those 'do it yourself' medicines the government hopes we'll one day kill ourselves with.

On one pre-season trip we were debriefed in the club's canteen, as I recall. The physio takes to the stage – there was no stage, just an expanse of floor – and feathers his wings as only a man who knows something that nobody else knows can. And even though he knows that nobody overly gives a shit what he is about to say, he stands there like a shameless cock. Preening himself until the laughter subsides.

'Now then,' he says, 'you all have your own routines I know, in terms of sleeping patterns et cetera, but we haven't been away to this side of the world as a team before. It's going to be new to you, and most importantly you'll need to sleep if you're going to perform and train well.'

Silence.

'To that end, the doc has prescribed these heavy-duty sleeping tablets. They'll put you to sleep for the flight and make sure that you are fine for training once we touch down in Asia, providing you take them the moment we take off. Any questions?'

Five seconds . . . ten seconds . . .

Finally an Irish voice from the back: 'Dey won't make us drowsy will dey?'

APRIL

I think the approved medical phrase for what is happening at the club right now is 'squeaky bum time'. We have only half a dozen league games left. We are at the business end of the campaign. Almost every club in the land still has something to play for, whether that involves avoiding being dragged into a relegation battle, trying to win a league, getting into the play-offs or, in the Premier League, fighting for European places. There are some mid-table clubs who are safe and either can't or don't have the ambition of a higher standing, which must be bloody boring for them; club staff are already mentally winding down after another mediocre season. Where you finish mid-table is worth a lot of money but not so much that it sets the heart of the club pumping every match day.

Of course winning things is exciting, but in a perverse sort of way so is fighting to avoid relegation. When you survive it's like winning the league. Some staff are motivated by the dread of spending next season in a lower division. That has implications for everybody at a club but especially for those with real-world problems like mortgages and car repayments.

Just hoping to have a job next year is no way to wind down a season.

Some in the Championship will be celebrating automatic promotion, and looking forward to replacing a Premier League club that has been lying dead in the relegation waters for the last third of the season. Even the paddles-to-the-chest shock therapy of a new manager could do nothing for them. At other clubs in the Championship everybody is hoping for those play-offs. The killer, of course, is getting all the way to the final only to fall short. That is devastating and can destroy the summer break. Your working year runs late to allow for the excitement of the play-offs, and then you end up with nothing? (Nothing except your job, the staff at relegated clubs might point out.)

We are lucky enough still to be contending for the Premier League title and still to be alive in the Champions League. We're looking forward to experiencing the nerve-jangling atmosphere of a couple of huge European nights. Those massive games, especially the away leg (for me anyway), are something to relish amid the unremitting grind of league play. There's something about the overwhelming noise in a famous continental stadium on a big death-or-glory European night that stirs the blood even of a physio. Imagine what it's like as a player!

For us in the medical room, the pressure is ratcheted up a notch now as the priorities change. Unlike the rest of the season, where we are just working to get a player fit as soon as possible, now there is a fundamental deadline, a specific date a player must reach. Suspensions mean some players are not available so there is added pressure to get replacements fit in time.

Players are desperate to play in big games. They may never

come around again. They want to be available despite carrying injuries, and those with borderline issues will do anything to be fit for title-deciding games. Our job is to protect them from themselves.

What I don't like at this time of year is telling a player he has no chance of playing. A big game is a deadline for which everybody wants to be declared fit. I have had players in tears when they realize they won't be ready. They shed some tears when they pick up a suspension too, but I'm not the one who has to break the news there.

Usually the player slowly realizes that he is coming up short in the lead-up to the game. If it's a close call the player and manager will have to make a decision based on the risk we have highlighted for them. This is especially the case with quarter-finals or semi-finals where there is another game to consider pretty soon afterwards. You have to weigh up whether it is worth getting injured and potentially not making the semi or final.

Players are optimists. It's always a little easier to tell a player he should sit this one out if he is convinced that he is being 'saved' for the biggest games of all.

I've seen the other side at clubs where there is really nothing to play for in the listless last few weeks and it becomes difficult to get the players out on the training field. Some of them just cannot be bothered. They make more of the little injuries they've been carrying over the season just to avoid playing any more games. Those are the days when you just want to get away for your holiday and leave them to it. Give me the high-octane death-or-glory stuff any time.

*

287

Forgive me if you have spotted this trend already.

Players are sponsored by certain brands. Those companies dictate what they wear. Now is the time of year when those deals look most worthwhile. Huge games with massive global audiences heighten the interest in our players. This is the bang those companies hoped for when they paid out their buck.

Players' boots are the battlefield for brands. As a physio I have to shake my head at this point. Tut-tut. Not good.

Players are being asked to use their feet as billboards, and to change those billboards at the whim of manufacturers. But some players are as valuable as racehorses nowadays. And their tools are their feet. No racehorse owner would let a farrier stick any old pair of shoes on to his investment. At football clubs, boot manufacturers decide what goes on the feet of a player.

In the old days when it came to boots you had to have thick leather and six studs underneath. Patrick boots were the classic in this mould. Kevin Keegan was sponsored to wear them even before the rest of football knew that you could be paid for the sort of boots you wore. They were a Belgian brand, and Keegan did what he was paid for. He made them fashionable in England – the deal left more of a fashion legacy than his famous bubble perm – even though apparently he wrote later that he didn't fancy the boots too much himself and only wore them for the money.

Players will wear boots they don't really like, just for the money. Who knew?

When that became apparent, the big manufacturers were in the water like piranha coming off a diet. By the 1990s Patrick had given up on football. The idea they had come up with had killed them. Nike, Adidas, Puma and co. were battling for the hearts, minds and feet of the footballing universe, and pro players were the targets.

Now, instead of the comforting thick leather shield you have leather (or more commonly just plastic) that is light, almost transparent, mixtures of studs and moulds, and carved heel cups at the back which are digging into people's Achilles. I despair when a player comes in brandishing his new space-age clogs having been sent a dozen of them by his sponsor and told to wear them for the next game, only to realize that their Achilles hates the pressure of the heel tab at the back or the sole plate is too flexible for their foot and their toes hurt.

Adidas brought out a boot not long ago with no laces. Players were wearing them within a few days. They have to be seen in the new boot. That's the deal, even among the iconic rebels of football.

But their feet don't have time to adapt. Every foot is different, just like every face is different, but most players don't have bespoke boots fitted and designed for them. They get sent a box of size eights from the manufacturers and a note saying 'We are launching these, please wear them in all games'. They are the same boots they could buy in Sports Direct but they have their name and national flag embroidered on the side, thus satisfying both the players' egos and the folks back home where they come from.

Most people can cope with a slight change in footwear, but a top-class sportsman not getting a boot which is designed around a template of his foot accounting for all the bunions and toe deviations, hard skin and old fracture scars and calluses amazes me. A player will come in and it will turn out that a stud under the big toe is irritating the living daylights out of him when he runs, really grating on the bones (usually one of the sesamoids), which creates an inflammatory problem, because the stud is in a slightly different position to the one on the previous boot. Or one day they have a boot whose sole plate is hard and flat, the next week they are wearing something where the sole plate is like a wave machine. They hurt. They have gone from a rigid footplate to a boot that is highly flexible.

The sock boot, another recent trend, is bad for some players. The boot goes a right in around the ankle – and tendons hate compression. After a while it will hurt. If you have a tendon problem and something is digging in, it causes a new problem or aggravates an old one.

Contrary to popular wisdom, I've not seen any convincing evidence that blades cause ACL injuries. (Unlike the traditional, round, peg-like studs, these blades measure up to 3 centimetres in length and are shaped to contour the foot, providing better stability for the standing foot when kicking.) Players like moulds in training and studs in games, unless the training pitches are really soft or, as at the top clubs, they are identical to the stadium pitches. Change is the main thing that causes injuries. If you are playing on grass and then you're suddenly required to play on AstroTurf you won't have had time to adapt. Your feet and ankles need time.

And surfaces really do differ. Premier League grounds are all virtually the same, but in countries like Ukraine or the Scandinavian nations they play on AstroTurf a lot now. Sutton United's home cup games this year were played on AstroTurf. Some pitches are heavier than others. Players need a range of footwear in order to cope with different surfaces. Alternatively, they can change the stud lengths on their boots.

There are odd things about footballers' feet which manufacturers never consider. It is normal for somebody who plays, let's say, left-back and only kicks with his left foot to have a very flexible left ankle. His left knee ligament may also be a little looser. It is normal for a footballer's feet to be abnormal. They are the intensively used instruments of his trade.

Wearing the output of different brands as an expression of individuality was never a great idea, even back when Kevin Keegan was wearing boots he didn't much like. For footballers, maybe the most important part of their individuality is their feet.

Do they listen?

Excuse me. I need some me time. I just have to go away and beat my head on a brick wall for a while.

At this time of the year more than any other the media are just outside noise. Inside the bubble you hardly hear that noise unless you really want to.

If you shut out the media and just get on with the work then all big games will be the same – that's the aim, anyway. Players have their habits, routines and their circadian rhythms. Nothing should upset them. So when they are in the medical room they don't need us telling them that we came across a few juicy titbits about their lives when we were flicking through the papers or Instagram earlier.

You see the odd player disinterestedly reading a tabloid, but unless there is something personally hurtful written about him he takes it all with dangerously unhealthy doses of salt. And if there is a quote from him it might be just vaguely familiar because his agent texted it to him just before he leaked it to a hack.

None of it seems real.

We have a big European match looming but you have to remember the clubs and the players that get to these prestigious occasions are used to it. We have been lucky to go to our fair share of cup finals and decisive games. The players tend to take it in their stride. In the medical room we don't carry on like fanboys. We just do our job. If we win we will be happy, but we will do the job just the same. If we lose, ditto.

Obviously when games are important you do feel it, but you try to treat them like every other game. There is more intensity and atmosphere before the big matches, understandably, but it is vital to approach them in the same way you would any other. Too much focus on one game always has the potential to affect the team negatively should they lose: in that scenario, defeat in an important fixture means it will be all the more difficult to pick the players up again.

Still, on a big European night you come out of the tunnel and you can sense the electricity crackling in the air. If we get a goal, I catch up with the action on the big screen, watch the scorer and make sure everybody gets up from the celebration shenanigans in one piece.

When the final whistle blows of course you get a little carried away. You haven't played but these are the people you work with every day, the lads who trust you and are professional enough to know that the medical staff are a key part of getting them on to the field. You're together for ten months of the year. So of course you'll throw your hands up in the air and high-five a few people (the football equivalent of dad dancing). But even then you'll still keep an eye out for the guy limping off and maybe trying to hide it.

It's dangerous out there for physios too. Gary Lewin, physio for Arsenal and then England, once had to be carried from the field on a stretcher after injuring his ankle while celebrating when Daniel Sturridge scored an equalizing goal for England against Italy. Gary dislocated his ankle and his assistant Steve Kemp had to take over physio duties. (The joke was that Sturridge is so injury-prone he can even cause his physio to get injured.) Gary's cousin Colin, who took over at Arsenal when Gary left, was once hit by a coin thrown from the stands, which is ironic as the Arsenal physio job pays pretty well already.

Europe. Brexiteer or Remainer or Dissenter, you have to love the place sometimes. Yes it's another country and they do things differently there, but that's the joy. A couple of us got around the city today for a brief walk and soaked up the sights and happy sounds of horns blaring and fans singing. The sight of locals and home and away fans sitting at pavement tables drinking moderately in the spring sunshine seemed so civilized and positive. It's so different from the fraught atmosphere at so many games at home.

We carry a 1-0 advantage into this Champions League semifinal second leg. We also carry a suspension and two injuries, which were borderline. Those two players won't play. Not my call. The management see that we still have a chance of stealing the league if results go right in the next couple of matches. We'll keep these players back because they will be needed later.

Tonight we hope to score on the counter but mainly we need to park the bus.

The food here is as wonderful as its reputation but most top teams take their own chef, who travels out the day before. They do a great job sourcing familiar food or taking British-branded ketchup with them. They try to keep the food similar to what we have at home, but I do like it when the resident hotel chef gets his way and throws in a few local or national dishes to try.

The team usually trains in the late afternoon the day before the game, at the stadium. It was just a couple of hours after they arrived but the flight was brief and the training was routine, just to get comfortable with the stadium and the pitch.

While they were training, the kitman and I had time to set ourselves up and familiarize ourselves with the environment. I love it here but the kitman is a stickler for making sure all the locks work so that the kit doesn't get stolen overnight. I leave those negotiations to him. You'll be surprised what goes missing. A food blender, used for making recovery drinks, and the stereo system (with extension lead) went AWOL once. No one touched the players' shirts.

After training it was dinner and more treatment for players, and massages for those wanting it. We worked late. It was past one in the morning when we got to lock up the hotel room we have been using as a temporary medical centre. Then it was time for a swift beer in the bar.

These trips can be knackering but it's important to stay upbeat. The players are tense enough as it is. I think hanging around the medical room becomes a source of normality. If we are just doing our jobs in the usual way and cracking the usual jokes it helps to keep their minds from racing, particularly the young guys who have never been on a stage this big before.

Our body clocks are only an hour ahead but bored players tend to notice the change and to feel their niggles a little bit more, and they request treatment – the sort of treatment they wouldn't request if the game was at home and they were lounging on their own sofas. When they aren't training or being treated they like to sleep. So they say. I often think they must have developed the ability to tweet and listen to music on headphones while getting some shut-eye.

Match day is much like any away game in England, except tonight's match is one of those that will determine how we remember this season. There's an optional breakfast for those not wanting a lie-in, then a walk and stretch (or a mini training session) before lunch, and a chance to sleep again in the afternoon. It's a perfect time for the physios to treat a few of the minor injuries.

Sometimes the build-up is worse than that. A lot of games in eastern Europe can be two to three hours ahead of UK time, with the game kicking off at ten p.m. local time. I'd be lying if I didn't hide the occasional yawn on the bench, hoping the TV cameras won't pick up my exhaustion (or boredom).

When you win or lose on nights like this there are always a few emotional minutes of aftermath chaos. The players linger on the pitch sharing their moment, good or bad, with the fans while we scuttle down the tunnel to get ready for our post-match chores. The players drift in after a while. As a group, as a club, this is our time together.

*

A late goal killed us tonight, but the boys were heroic. There are no medals on offer for heroism though. When we win there's lots of whooping and shouting and then, yes, it gets boring. It's business as usual. Treat the injured, tidy up, pack away, get a shower. Tonight we lost and it's the same routine as if we had won, it's just that we have a different theme song.

A few words are spoken by the manager. The players are quiet. We speak to each other softly as if somebody has passed away. We get things done quickly and then we get ready to get out of there. After the game, everyone just wants to get on that plane as soon as possible. If we win, players may warm down (not often, though); those who haven't played may run around like headless chickens for fifteen to twenty minutes, trying to justify having a day off the following day. Tonight, everyone just wants to get home.

Doping control takes an age, as usual. Having played ninety minutes, players can take up to two hours to produce a urine sample copious enough for testing (it's not a lot really, but still hard to produce on demand). Players hate being picked out for random testing at the best of times because they know that, having held everyone up, they won't be popular on the way home. I always pray for them to pull the substitutes out of the hat. That didn't happen tonight, and the two players sat together silent and solemn in the medical room as if they were attending the post-mortem of a loved one.

People say to me when the season ends, 'Oooh, I bet you'll miss it. All the excitement is over – you won't know what to do with yourself.' Never. Nights like tonight, even as a physio, are a build-up of excitement and tension. You stay detached, do the things you always do, but you would need to be a robot not to have a sense of the occasion and what it means. You see lines you've never noticed before on the faces of the coaching staff. You hear new expletives. You see new heroes being created and older players' expiry dates being examined. Some of them will never know another night like this. You love it all madly, but the break that is now coming into view over the brow of the hill will be wonderful.

TSF: Second Opinion

You never know who is out to kill you

Every footballer has his own diet. And every footballer has his one staple dish. The dish he cooks in his own home, away from the training ground and the chef's boiled brown rice, steamed broccoli and plain chicken breast with no seasoning and the skin removed.

With all the people dying of hunger in the world it seems a little churlish to moan about having plenty to eat. The real issue here is flavour. Trying to inject flavour into a diet as severe as a footballer's is a problem on a par with trying to solve North Korea.

I achieved the impossible like so:

- One bag of dried penne pasta
- One jar of Loyd Grossman tomato and roasted garlic sauce
- Pinch of salt
- Olive oil

I give you the dish that I ate every single day for the best part of fifteen years. Boil the kettle and tip the water on to the pasta to speed up the cooking, sieve out the lumps of tomato in the sauce thus achieving a smooth consistency, add a pinch of salt at the end and a splash of good olive oil.

What can possibly go wrong?

The day started like any other. Match day. Up at nine a.m. (never lie in, you'll be fucked when three p.m. comes around). Start sipping water immediately from a 2-litre bottle. Wait until eleven, then start cooking. But that day the pasta tasted strange. Believe me, after a number of years of perfecting the dish, including the exact cooking time of the pasta (six minutes and forty-five seconds), I know how it should taste. Nonetheless, there was no more pasta so I wolfed it down and carried on sipping water.

Interestingly, that water re-emerged a few hours later from a different place in an eye-catching new shade, the sort that would have very charmingly decorated the walls of homes in 1970s Britain. But this was 2008, and in the twenty-first century that same colour screams trouble.

I got to the stadium and rushed past everybody asking for autographs. Both of them. I made it to trap one, as we footballers call the bogs, and downloaded a stream of data Google would have struggled to fit on to its servers.

The physio poked his head around the corner and probably wished he hadn't.

'Everything all right?'

I have perfected a look over the years that I give people who ask me stupid questions. Mostly journalists. Still, I had to see the physio every day and it was his job to help me so he got an answer.

'Oddly enough, phys, I am *not* all right.'

He gave me Gaviscon, paracetamol and antacid. When three points are on the line it is paramount to give a player as many legal drugs as possible to get him through the game and then deal with the morgue and the next of kin at the appropriate juncture thereafter.

I made it through the game, which we won, and better still I made it back to the house just in time to test out how seventies décor looks in a nice modern bathroom. Semi-relaxed, I slunk into the lounge and put the telly on while I waited to die.

Mrs TSF came in and I explained why she should not get too close. I didn't know at that point whether it was a bug I might pass on to her. She dealt with it in her own unique style.

'Do you want a cup of tea?' she asked.

'No, I don't want anything that's brown.'

'I'll make you a tea anyway.'

She wandered off to the kitchen.

'What happened to the water that was in this kettle?' she shouted back to me.

'I used it on my pasta,' I shouted back.

Mrs TSF slowly walked back into the lounge and stared at me.

'What?' I asked.

'You used that water for your pasta? It had kettle descaler in it. I left it overnight and meant to clean it out this morning.'

My own wife! Mind you, if she had succeeded in killing me we'd both be a lot richer than we are now. Bloody amateur.

The sanctuary of the physio room

At most clubs the physio room is bolted on to the changing room. Despite the fact that the rules of bullying younger players have changed, this is still a problem for the modern-day youth-team player.

I have seen youth-team players who have been instructed to get the manager something from the first-team dressing room standing on the other side of the door almost in tears at the prospect of entering. The moment they walk in, the most senior players tend to grab them before making them tell the squad everything about their girlfriends, humiliating their general knowledge and then getting them to sing a couple of songs. At least that's how it used to be. Most youth-team players are bulletproof these days. But every now and then the most timid players are set upon by the baying pack.

That said, there are moments when the senior squad give over the changing room to the youth team so they can play their Tuesday night FA Cup matches. The first team are encouraged to come along to the later rounds if the team has progressed that far. For many of the youth-team players it is as far as their career will ever go, so it's a show of support that sends out the message that we're all here for one another rather than offering up the reality, which is that of a bunch of mercenaries.

I have the distinct recollection of youth-team matches being played at night under floodlights in the numbing cold, and as such the physio room became a sanctuary for first-team players who were freezing their bollocks off and seeking a warm drink at half-time. The players would cram in five minutes before the youth team came into the changing room for their half-time team talk. At that particular club there was one door into the changing room, and as such the physio room too. Once you were in, you were trapped and reduced to whispering until the buzzer went.

A quick sidestep here: unused first-team players also like to do this when first teams are losing so that they can hear every word of the manager's bollockings. It's the only perk of being an unused squad player.

The youth team were losing. Their manager was not happy. But the first-team manager was unhappier still. We were huddled into the physio room around two minutes into the youth-team manager's rant when we heard an almighty bang. As players who had been on the end of hammerings ourselves we were hard-wired to recognize that the bang was the changing-room door being removed from its hinges.

It was the first-team manager.

'What the fuck was that?' he screamed. 'Three-nil? It should never be a three-nil game! It's only a three-nil game because you've allowed it to be!'

Already had the makings of a classic.

'Right, you! Stop letting the fucking winger come inside, show him down the line – it's fucking basic stuff!'

Muffled laughter in the physio room . . .

'You! Any chance of making a tackle? It's the biggest game you're ever gonna play in if you don't pull your head out of your arse!'

Snorts and giggles from the physio room . . .

'Striker, the goal is the white thing at the end of the pitch. See the goalposts? Fucking stay in between them! And another thing . . . when I marked Pelé he didn't once control the ball with the outside of his fucking foot! If I see you try to control the ball like that again you can fuck off out of this club!'

A bunch of first-team players with their hands over their mouths trying not to burst out laughing . . .

'Right, play with some fucking pride and win the second half! You can all fuck off outside and wait for them to come out, but do you all understand what I've said? Any fucking questions?'

Bated breath in the physio room . . .

I was told later that the striker had raised his hand before asking his question. Never raise your hand before asking a question – and never, for the love of God, ask a question.

'WHAT?!' screamed the manager.

The striker looked around nervously.

'Who's Pelé?'

The physio room fell apart that evening.

Nuts!

Life was tough when I played football as a fresh-faced sixteen-year-old kid. I was a late starter in so many ways. I didn't go through a youth team and I didn't talk to a girl in earnest until I was about eighteen. I tell myself it was because I was taking my football extremely seriously. The reality is I was shy and in awe of my friends, who found talking to girls as easy as they would find slipping into a post-school life of alcohol, Benidorm and 2.4 kids at the expense of the prom queen.

Although, I may still be bitter.

This all ties in with my first real injury, so stay with me.

I was playing for the youth team of a reputable non-league side and it was at a time when cocky kids were becoming men. And at that point in adolescence, nature really begins to weed out the weak. It turns out that I was weak. In terms of football, the tackles become a bit more crunching. Players become a bit faster than others, talking on the pitch turns to sledging and swearing, and fair play turns into a will to win that is not afraid to overstep the mark and intimidate the pea hearts.

I wasn't at the top of the food chain, but I wasn't at the bottom either. I didn't mind swearing or being physical. I didn't mind squaring up, although that was rare, and I didn't mind going in for a tackle.

But as with most things in adolescence, there is a learning curve. You learn how not to offend women when you talk to them. You learn how to strike down an opponent with a well-placed acid drop. You learn how to fight. And you learn when to go in for a tackle and when not to.

And some people have more outrageous stories about their learning curve than others.

The ball broke between myself and somebody I weighed up to be of a similar stature and ripe for a bit of chest-beating once I'd inevitably won the ball and pushed his face into the mud. We both slid in – I've since learned to stand up – and our legs managed to miss the ball while our momentum took us hurtling towards each other's nether regions.

I came off worse.

In the hospital, the surgeon explained that it was a simple

case of pushing the testicle back into the sack and sewing it up. But first he'd have to drain the fluid that had accrued in the region.

Do what you have to do, Doc.

'Just one more thing,' he said. 'Do you mind if a couple of graduates stand in to learn about this procedure? It's quite an interesting and unusual operation.'

And if I say no?

'Great, this is Jenny and Olivia.'

Fuck. This happened at a time in my life when Victorian nudie shots would give a kid a hard-on.

'Nice to meet you,' I said, looking at the ceiling.

I lost my inhibitions that day, and all it took was a severed bollock. I figured that two very attractive women had seen my special place and that meant that I was no longer a virgin. Today I have a lovely thin white scar running around my nut sack and when women ask I am no longer embarrassed. I treat my rite of passage as something of a conversation piece.

The longest in the shower

People often wonder why there aren't as many female physios in the game as there perhaps should be.

I have worked with female physios and masseuses too. The problem is not with the women. The problem is with our own physical perfection. And our notions about it. Yes, it's tough being an Adonis. Don't knock it till you've tried it.

Many players are toned to within an inch of their life and

some women simply can't apply the pressure to an area that is needed to ease the tension in the muscle.

Stop sniggering at the back.

It goes two ways – like some footballers I know. Most footballers are at ease with changing in front of anyone. We've been getting changed in front of people since we were kids, but we'll let the tribunal deal with that. Nudity doesn't have the same effect on us as it does on mere mortals. Peter Crouch once said, if he hadn't been a footballer, he'd have been a virgin, but he's an exception.

I'm just ripped and buff. And I hardly notice. We fear nobody in that sense.

But occasionally you have a bad game. You are soundly beaten. It's been a freezing cold night in Stoke and the morale is as low as the temperature. The crowd has been ragging on you from the first whistle. And you have missed an open goal – something I never did, of course; this is a hypothetical scenario I am painting.

Maybe you were at fault for one of their goals when you let your man go from a set-piece. The manager has torn a strip off you afterwards and generally you feel about as cut up as you can get. Your feet are so cold you wonder if you will ever feel them again.

But this is football and we can always go a little bit lower.

The manager finishes his rant. He storms off to drink a convivial glass of wine with his victorious opposite number. One or two of the players start to move. The captain says, 'Come on lads, aye, let's get on the fucking bus and get out of here.' People begin to change. The physios start packing up their tables and bags.

The lads head to the shower. You still feel like a piece of frozen shit and you just wish you were at home.

You notice in your misery that your poor penis has shrunk to the size of a baby prawn. Absentmindedly you begin to jig it a little. Come on, for fuck's sake, it's not that bad. At least make some effort. No, nothing. You are cold and miserable and your cock is hiding.

Just then you glance up and meet the eyes of the female physio. Only her eyes don't meet yours. She's looking at your privates and marvelling at the workmanship involved in producing replica genitalia in miniature.

You've had a great working relationship with her up to this point. But that's pity you see in her eyes for just that moment.

She quickly looks away and goes about her business. She is a professional. You go to comment to the player standing next to you about what's just happened, only to realize that he is the captain of Nigeria. On your other side is the national goalkeeper for Ghana.

Football is a fucking rubbish game sometimes and some stereotypes are just hurtful on many levels.

MAY

It is bright and sunny when I arrive at the training ground. I have come here in darkness, in fog, in sleet, in rain and in despair during the course of this season. I have come here jaded on the mornings after away games in our Champions League run, and I've waited for the players to arrive and the buzz from the previous night to transfuse us all and banish the tiredness. I have come here disappointed on the morning after it was mathematically certain we weren't going to win the league. And I can't think of a day that I didn't enjoy. My job is the same, win or lose, but I grow attached to the staff and players as individuals and as a group. I keep my clinical distance, but the part of me that loves the job says that we are all in it together. And we are.

When players come in to see us with injuries and knocks it is not because they want to be in the physio room instead of training. This is their career, and it is short. So we lift them up, keep them happy and focused, talk with them, find the human connection, build the trust.

It's impossible not to root for those guys on a Saturday afternoon or a Wednesday night.

Throughout the season my day at the training ground has always started around 8.30 a.m., with a medical meeting to discuss the 'current' plan for the day. Then a meeting with the coaching staff to update them of any medical issues. Fit players tend to start drifting in at around ten, half an hour before training.

Once you throw players into the mix, the best-laid plans of coaches and physios go out the window. I'm not sure any longer why we even have those early-morning planning meetings.

This news may shock you, but footballers don't really appreciate the implications of their actions. How often this year have I had a player stroll into the medical room thirty minutes before training starts and announce that his knee hurts and he can't train? Or, worse, he just can't put his finger on it but he doesn't feel right or proper?

It is a nightmare. Not for the player, for me. My day invariably sounded good when I unfolded it at the planning meeting.

Coaches hate last-minute changes more than I do. They meticulously prepare the training for the day – well, most of them – and suddenly having to pull a player out half an hour or so before it starts makes them mad. The player numbers change and they have to 'borrow' one from the reserve or youth squad, which then affects their session accordingly.

I've known some players who have fallen out with the manager and they will ring each other in their cars on the way to training to discuss whether they are going to train just to annoy the manager or to fake a particular injury to get out of training altogether.

In all these turf wars I am an innocent bystander, insisting on my neutrality.

I've had managers make me keep players at the training ground until seven p.m. because the manager thought the player was malingering. He wanted to mess the player's day up. My day didn't matter.

Still neutral.

Some mornings everything changes due to a new issue like a player texting that he has woken up with an illness or a stiff back. Or, as in the case of Ross McCormack at Villa this year, he breaks the bad news that the gate to his gated community is stuck and he's imprisoned. A sick player has to be visited by a doctor – you don't want contagious players around the training ground – and has to notify the coaching staff that the planned training session must change. A player tragically trapped at home can expect a drive-by from an angry manager.

What I have always liked is that every day is different. The rhythm is dictated by the games and the players. Training days and days off are planned around when we play. The mood goes up and down with the results.

In an ideal world, the training schedule – start times, travel arrangements, etc. – for the month ahead would be produced in the last week of the previous month. I have never really worked in an ideal world. Thankfully. It must be very boring there.

I have seen dumb coaches who think it is smart to punish players for a lacklustre performance by driving them harder and harder for the next couple of days. That just guarantees a tired, resentful performance next time out. I've seen coaches who have bored players catatonic with the grinding repetitiveness of their sessions. The monotony has been the message.

This year, though, I have seen enlightened, inventive sessions where the mood is easy and the players are enjoying themselves just enough that they forget to grumble. I have seen a management team that likes to talk. They are infectious. Those things that fans and pundits never see make for a better place to work.

But if you're winning it makes the pain less noticeable. Also, players want to play and not lose their place in the squad. Remember, the more football you play, the better you are to play football.

I have loved the training-ground days, but match days give you a buzz, so long as you don't end up doing sixty to seventy games a year. Then the games tend to just meld into one another in my memory. Fans remember great goals. I remember interesting injuries.

Somehow this season I have managed to fit a family life into all of this. I have learned to nod my head and smile when people tell me how lucky I am to have the entire summer off every year – because of course all player injuries clear themselves up in mid-May.

The season is now dwindling fast. We have a dead-rubber home game to finish but it's a chance for the players to applaud the crowd and thank them for their support this season, and vice versa. Then they'll be away, scattering themselves and their money across the world. I'll be here mostly, just quietly worrying about which striker will injure himself in a jet ski accident or which goalie will drop a bottle of salad cream on his foot with disastrous consequences.

May they not get injured, but if they do, may their injuries be interesting.

A football writer once said to me that to be good at his job he needed to care about the writing part more than he cared about the football part. It was the most sensible thing I have ever heard a football writer come out with. It's the same with being a sports physio. You need to love being a physio more than you love the sport you work in. Don't be a fan with a physio bag.

I like football and footballers, but I don't love either. I don't consider myself a diehard fan. When people want to bend my ear about the formation the club is playing or what I think of their theories about this player or that, I lose the will to live fairly quickly.

To be honest, overseeing games is not such a challenge. All you are doing on match day is prepping players who are essentially fit and administering first aid to those who pick up an injury. If you give me an injury that isn't getting better or somebody who wants to be fit in three months' time instead of four, that to me is a challenge. Strapping an ankle or giving a hamstring a rub? Not so much. After that work is done I'm half hoping that somebody might get an injury during the game, just so that I have something stimulating to do.

Yeah. Dirty little secret. I get excited when a player goes down. It gives me a bit of a thrill. I can contribute. I'm not sitting there with my voodoo dolls willing players to get injured, you understand, but as injuries are going to happen anyway . . . If I am good at my job in that pressure situation then I have made a difference. If you have a busy day it's because you've had lots of injuries. For the team, a physio with nothing to do is good news. But not necessarily for the physio. Generally, a successful medical team is a bored medical team. You should have nothing to do. But injuries are what it's all about from a career point of view.

Serious head injuries or heart attacks are at the outer limit of what we expect to encounter in an average working day, but we have to be ready for them too. The same applies for the gruesome injuries. You're not much use to anybody if you run on to the field, find that the centre-half's tibia is sticking out through his skin and there is blood everywhere, and all you can do is mutter phrases like 'Oh no!' and 'Shit, I think I want to be sick,' as one physio I worked with said when covering a reserve game. It didn't give the player much confidence.

In the Premier League, probably the most famous injury in terms of its horror was what happened to David Busst of Coventry just eighty-seven seconds into a league match at Old Trafford in April 1996. He challenged for a ball between Denis Irwin and Brian McClair, encountered two physical forces coming from different directions, and suffered extensive compound fractures to both the tibia and fibula of his right leg. After the collision his shin stuck out from his lower leg like the prow of a shipwrecked vessel. There was blood everywhere. Peter Schmeichel, the United keeper, as solid a Viking as ever there was, is said to have thrown up in his own goal area. Schmeichel and several other players needed counselling afterwards.

It would be hard to say that Busst was lucky. He ended up needing twenty-six operations, catching MRSA, and never playing again. I remember reading a few years ago a piece in which he said he was slightly fortunate in that the injury had occurred at Old Trafford. He was tended to by medics from both teams and – something that was rare enough in those days – there was easy access for an ambulance to come straight on to the field. 'But Man United have the biggest speed bumps outside their ground,' he continued. 'I was on gas and air at that time and it wasn't helping whatsoever. Up, down, up, down. That was the funny thing about it.'

We can't get everything right.

Although Busst's injury is imprinted in the minds of all football people old enough to remember it, sport has thrown up worse injuries and more dangerous situations.

Imagine being a fan with a physio bag in Buffalo back in March 1989 during the ice hockey game between the St Louis Blues and the Buffalo Sabres. There was a hard collision between a player from either side in front of the Buffalo goal crease. Steve Tuttle, the attacking player for St Louis, and Uwe Krupp, the Buffalo defender, upended each other and crashed into the goal area. Tuttle's skate blade slashed across the neck of the Buffalo goaltender Clint Malarchuk, severing his carotid artery and injuring the surrounding sheath muscle and jugular vein.

A geyser of blood spurted from Malarchuk's neck, pooling vividly on the pristine ice. Three players and many spectators vomited, eleven fans fainted and two suffered a cardiac arrest as, in an all-too-clear rhythm, every time Malarchuk's heart struck a beat, the blood issued energetically from his neck. TV went to commercials. Meanwhile Malarchuk, who was dying but keenly aware as people are in these moments of something odd, was concerned that his mother was watching the game live on television.

As people stood and gaped in horror a guy called Jim Pizzutelli, a trainer on the Buffalo bench who had formerly been a medic in Vietnam, skated over to the goaltender. Pizzutelli calmly reached into Malarchuk's neck and pinched off the bleeding with his thumb and forefinger. He then assisted him from the ice at the player's request (still thinking about his mother). As luck would have it, Buffalo were defending the end where the dressing rooms were and the exit was behind Malarchuk's goal.

In the dressing room, the team doctor applied extreme pressure to the wound by kneeling on the goalie's collarbone. The procedure, calculated to produce a low breathing rate and low metabolic state, is most uncomfortable, but when asked, most people judge it to be a preferable alternative to bleeding to death.

The doctor suggested to Malarchuk that he let him know whenever he needed a breath. Malarchuk would wince in distress and the doctor would relieve the pressure momentarily and the blood would spurt. This grotesque embrace continued in the ambulance all the way to Buffalo General Hospital.

By the time the medics were finished, Clint Malarchuk had lost a litre and a half of blood and it had taken three hundred stitches to staunch the wound.

Sometimes the only thing separating any of us from tragedy

is the ultimate good luck of having somebody well trained and clinically detached nearby. Fabrice Muamba regularly commends the Bolton doctor Jonathan Tobin for his expertise. Without him and his staff, Fabrice would not have survived his cardiac arrest.

As a postscript, Clint Malarchuk, who was dogged all his life by depression and OCD issues, played lower-league hockey for a couple more years and continued his association with the game in retirement. In 2008 he attempted to blow his brains out with a rifle. The bullet is still lodged in his head but he survived.

Sometimes things are just meant to be.

There was a story a couple of years back from the Ukrainian Premier League where one player saved the life of another.

The Dynamo Kiev captain Oleg Gusev was involved in a collision with the Dnipro goalkeeper Denys Boyko. Gusev was knocked unconscious after the keeper's knee hit him in the face, which caused him to swallow his tongue, blocking his airway and making it difficult for him to breathe.

The Dnipro midfielder Jaba Kankava saved the day. Kankava forced his hand down Gusev's throat and freed the tongue, allowing Gusev to breathe properly again. For his trouble, Kankava got bitten in the process.

To stop somebody from 'swallowing' their tongue you don't have to reach into their mouth. Indeed it is better not to. But Gusev had broken his jaw. With the jaw 'unattached', the tongue had fallen back and blocked the airway. Usually in these situations where there isn't a broken jaw or something in the mouth like a mouthguard, the best action is simply to put your fingers behind the jaw and gently push it forward to open the airway – technically called a 'jaw thrust'. Or if there is no indication of neck injury, just perform a 'head tilt, chin lift' manoeuvre. That simple process uses gravity to let the tongue fall forward again and open the airway. Just push on the angle of the jaw and tilt the head gently forwards. This is also useful if you need to get access to the mouth for other reasons.

(Because in reality, you don't actually 'swallow your tongue'. When you are unconscious, the soft palate – the tissue that the tongue is connected to – becomes relaxed and falls to the back of the throat, thus blocking the airway.)

It was an amazing feat for a player to be alert enough to pick up the signs of an unconscious player not breathing. Most players are oblivious to the severity of head injuries and haven't got a clue what to do when one occurs near them. I have been involved in a few serious head injury incidents and players just stand around looking helpless, or they do the opposite and try to be heroes. But they can do more harm than good, or just get in the way of the trained medical staff.

When a player is knocked out, he becomes completely flaccid, either due to the impact from the initial collision with another player or from wrenching the backbone when he hit the deck. He may have sustained a spinal injury so the spine has to be protected. Hence you see the medics, when they run on to the pitch, going straight to the head and holding it. Although protecting the spine is important, they must ensure that the basic signs of life – airway, breathing, circulation – are present. The player's ability to breathe and circulate blood is fundamental. There is no point protecting someone's neck if they aren't breathing. 'The good news is we protected your loved one's neck. The bad news is . . .' Nobody wants to make that call.

It's a stressful situation, but medical staff are trained to a high level these days and go into automatic pilot mode, oblivious to the crowd and what is around them, in order to deal with the player effectively.

Every player in every league should be able to do what Jaba Kankava did, however. Just not in the way he did it. Unless you want to lose a finger.

Do you remember the movie *The Island*? Ewan McGregor? Not many people do. It got such a quiet reception in 2005 that it seemed more like an islet than an island. The premise was that in 2019 the very rich would have clones living in a massive compound that would basically serve as an Argos store. If you found yourself injured or ill, the replacement parts you needed to regain health would be harvested from your clone.

Of course the clones had to be told a nice story to keep them happy in the oppressive compound where they actually lived miserable lives. They believed that the entire outside world was contaminated and they were in the domed compound for their own protection.

Once a week in the compound a lottery would be held. The winner, it was believed, would get to leave the compound and go to live on the one contagion-free island still left in the world. Paradise. The snag was, there was no such island. The winner was just being taken away so that their parts could be used for organ harvesting, surrogate motherhood and other purposes to benefit each clone's sponsor – the rich person who was identical to them in appearance.

In the end, Ewan McGregor makes everything better.

In a mixed-up way, *The Island* might just have provided a vision of the future of sports medicine. We only have to unscramble the plot and change it around a bit. Obviously it's the world's greatest sports stars who actually believe that the outside world is contaminated, but go with me on this. While those stars' employers would happily create compounds full of clones in order to prolong their stars' careers, we may already have jumped ahead of all that with regenerative medicine.

Custom-made living body parts have already been produced using 3D printers. The sections of bone, muscle and cartilage all functioned normally when implanted into animals. The technology is moving quickly towards the stage where scientists believe they will be able to replicate living tissues in order to repair the human body.

Until recently the limit on progress was set at the seemingly impossible task of keeping cells alive. Cells were quickly starved of oxygen and nutrients in tissues thicker than 0.2 millimetres. At Wake Forest Baptist Medical Center a new technique was developed that 3D-prints a tissue riddled with micro-channels, rather like a sponge, to allow nutrients to penetrate the tissue. The Integrated Tissue and Organ Printing System (or Itop) uses a mixture of biodegradable plastic (to provide the structure) and a water-based gel to provide the cells and encourages them to grow.

When these structures were implanted into animals, the plastic broke down as it was replaced by a natural, structural 'matrix' of proteins produced by the cells. Meanwhile, blood vessels and nerves grew into the implants.

They are now ready to print body parts on a human scale.

The science of bioprinting isn't even twenty years old. Extraordinary to think that somebody discovered that living cells could be sprayed through the nozzles of inkjet printers and kept intact. That must have livened up a dull day at the office.

Now that we (all right, not me) are able to use printers to generate different cell types and the polymers that provide a scaffold that helps keep the structure in shape, it will be possible to deposit layer upon layer of cells that will bind together and grow into living, functional tissue. Scientists are already experimenting with kidney and liver tissue, skin, bones and cartilage. They are implanting printed ears, bones and muscles into animals. These integrate properly with their hosts. At Northwestern University in Chicago they printed working prosthetic ovaries for mice. The recipients were able to conceive and give birth.

Now, if a mouse can get prosthetic ovaries, how long will it be before Ronaldo is getting new cartilage or new muscle tissue? Ronaldo Inc. has way more money than a mouse. Ronaldo Inc. has way more money than most of the struggling people the science is designed to help.

Modern players are so specifically suited to their positions that in terms of the physical specimens they represent they are almost clones of each other already. Watch top players get off the coach and you can usually tell who plays where. And certain injuries follow certain positions. Wingers get hamstring injuries. Goalkeepers or centre-halves get patellar tendon problems. From now to a day when we have a ready-made supply of the right cartilages and ligaments for repair work isn't a big jump.

Rival pharmaceutical companies and businesses pushing 3D biological treatments will be barging each other out of the way to get a piece of this market. I see them using players to sell these things. A fifty-six-year-old Ronaldo saying that he has never felt better since he got his new X7 knee from Tissue Regenerative Systems, the one-stop shop for new body parts. When Lionel Messi wants a meniscus, where does he go? That's right . . .

In another season we could even have pulled off a Leicester City and won the league, but ultimately we fell well short. We'd have taken that at the start of the year, thank you very much.

At lunch today we were talking about what that means on the bottom line. For the next three years the domestic TV rights for the Premier League are worth £5.136 billion. Throw in the overseas rights and the total reaches about £8 billion. Each year 50 per cent of the annual TV rights gets divided equally between all the Premier League clubs. So we get £38 million this year. Twenty-five per cent gets divided according to how you finished. We're going to get another £38 million based on our final position in the table (the champions get £2 million more). Facility fees for being live on the telly will bring us £23 million. Money from overseas rights will be divided equally too, giving us £48 million more.

That's £147 million, basically, for just being on the telly. That's before we sold a ticket, a corporate box, a few shirts and hats, or a halfway decent player to China. It's before you count our shirt sponsorship deal, our main sponsors and our Noah's ark full of 'official partners' (domestic and overseas, one of each). It's before we look at the Champions League revenue, which we have secured once again for next year. It's before we sell a match programme or a meat pie or a stadium tour or a parking spot.

We're doing OK, we decided.

But at the lunch table we were all medical room nerds. We're not happy.

The Premier League is so rich you would imagine that it surely must be at the cutting edge of every piece of injury-related technology and innovation. Not true, but I know why people would imagine that. You look at the wage bill of a Premier League club and how many millions of pounds' worth of working days are lost through player injuries in the course of a season and it is blindingly obvious that it would be in the interest of football to get out front in terms of doing our own research. We could pool resources to get a university to do it. We could do as the Swedes do and join forces with government to research sports injuries on the basis that much of what we learn would be of use to the general population too.

Sadly, when it comes to research, clubs are all but useless at instigating and implementing studies. You can't experiment on players, obviously, so we just piggyback on the work of others. We use the resources of research bodies and academic institutions and other leagues in other sports.

I look at players now and I agree that we look after them a lot better than we used to. There is more appreciation that the guys must have a life after football. Materially, an average league player's best aim for his career is to have his house paid off when his playing days end. All else is gravy. We have kids in the academy and they are good kids, sixteen or seventeen years old. But they are on amazing money for kids of that age and they are spending thousands of pounds in nightclubs buying champagne. We can't give them common-sense transfusions.

I am amazed constantly by the stories of lads who earned enough to last two lifetimes but who find themselves in money trouble. Check out the book *Retired* by Alan Gernon. It contains many scary stories and statistics of what happens to footballers when they finish playing. Every player should read it.

Spiritually and physically, a player should end his career in good condition and be expecting a healthy and happy life. But a lot of players suffer badly in the transition into retirement. They miss the exercise, the competitiveness, the adrenalin, the company, the routine, the attention. Rates of depression, addiction, bankruptcy and marriage break-up are distressingly high for this group.

When it comes to physical health for retiring players we have changed our approach more effectively, I think. Most players should be able to kick a football around with their grandkids at some stage down the road. We have more knowledge now of care and due diligence. We look at the bigger picture and longer story, usually for more time than the club appreciates. The club wants the player to be well for the next three years. Ideally, when those three years are up the club would like to be able to say to another club that, yes, he has a lot of mileage on the clock, but if you buy him you should find him reliable enough.

That seems short term, and out there in the real world it is. For a football club even to be considering what may happen a year or two down the road is a miracle. We work in the culture of the next game, the next session, the next ball.

We have improved. But we need to do better.

I don't mind if physios and doctors get taken for granted in a football club. In the background, not in the limelight. We are background staff. It is not about us, and if we don't like the pressure or if we are envious of the limelight we can always go and work in the general community. I don't think, though, that players or their clubs understand how seriously we now take the long-term welfare of the player and how much protection our more modern approach offers to clubs against legal action.

What if all the old ex-players, bandy-legged and limping in and out of hospitals getting new hips and new knees, were to sit down with gimlet-eyed lawyers who would go on to ask their former clubs to explain why players were once routinely pumped with cortisone to get them through games and seasons? I think there would be some uncomfortable conversations and shockwaves of litigation.

That isn't in our culture yet. The players carry the wounds of war as stoically as they carry the knowledge that back in the day they played in front of huge attendances every week but the money went into the pockets of directors and chairmen. That was just the way football worked. But there will come a time when players will be encouraged to litigate against the football industry if they carry a legacy of injury into middle age and beyond.

The way football works has changed now, and players' views of the care given to them during their professional lives is changing too. I think we owe it to ourselves, the players and to the general medical services who lack the finances we possess to be a bit more proactive about research into treatments and the business of avoiding injuries – prevention strategies, or 'prehab' as we like to call it now.

I know of one leading Premier League club that has no sports scientist employed with the first team and no GPS monitoring system is used with their players. It is left to the experience of the coaching staff to ensure that the intensity of the players' training is at its optimal level.

My bet is that sports science is reaching its final frontiers faster than its cousin, medical science, is.

Ewan McGregor, your time will come.

Our time, or another season's worth of it, has passed. School's out.

It is so important for us to get a break from the game in the summer. We played so many games this season that at the moment they are just a big blob in my memory. Half of the games were on the road and I can't count the days and nights spent in hotels.

On average, a player will get at least one injury per season and will therefore get a period of time off the treadmill, but spare a thought for the backroom staff! We provide a seven-day-a-week service all year round.

These days, when the summer comes there are many reha-bilitation centres all over the world that we use to send players to in order that they can continue their rehab in a different environment. This breaks the monotony of going to the train-ing ground and gives the player an extra boost before returning in July. The most popular spots are in America, Italy, Qatar and Biarritz in France.

Surprised?

In the UK, there is a rehabilitation centre based at St George's Park near Burton, with places funded by the Professional Footballers' Association. The players are residents and undergo intensive treatment. Sessions last all day, Monday to Friday. I have sent players there and many get fed up after a few days, although there is a nice pub a few miles away that keeps some of them happy. And while I'm away with the family, I don't worry about them too much.

I'd rather go somewhere warmer though, wouldn't you?

Family life does take a terrible beating when you work in football. You may get a day off during the week, when the wife is at work – yes, not all wives are WAGs spending their time shopping and in spas – and the kids are at school, to catch up on 'home life'. I'm usually faced with a list of chores when I get a day off. But I can't complain about that. I am away for the majority of the weekends, especially now that many games are on Saturdays and Sundays, and, this season, Monday and Friday nights. No day is safe any more. What with training on a Saturday morning, then a hotel in the evening before the game the following day, I've very much become a non-weekend dad.

After the last game of the season I got home late. My wife was fast asleep. The kids were deep in their dreams when I checked in on them. Most of our time together as a family during the season is spent sleeping.

I'm used to getting home when everyone is in bed. My other half understands the job by now.

In the mornings, over breakfast, I do sound off about the frustrating things such as annoying colleagues and stupid club decisions, but most of the time I tend not to talk about the detail much. My wife finds it boring and the kids suddenly get very interested in getting to school.

And I probably take some of it for granted. I must have covered a thousand football games by now, experiencing finals and relegation dogfights and dull dead-rubber matches, going to Wembley, the Bernabéu and other places that most people only have on their bucket lists. Sometimes I have to remind myself how lucky I am. But like any job it can get routine and dull.

I welcome the summer break now like a parched man welcomes chilled water. If anything I know that it will pass too quickly. The season is long and demanding, especially when you have family, so getting away from it all is going to be wonderful . . . and necessary.

As I sit reading a book near a pool with the kids playing and the missus soaking up the sun, a part of me will miss the noise of the medical room, the daily edition of drama and conse-quence. But the mobile will be close to hand, and I can't help but check it a few times a day in case there's a medical to do or someone needs something.

I often daydream about leaving football and going out to start my own practice, but I think that would prove dull. A conveyor belt of patient after patient every thirty minutes. I've come to realize that the club would have to sack me for reasons that weren't in any way my fault (too efficient about keeping records or something) and pay me off with enough money to buy two corporate boxes. But many physios have been a victim of this in the past.

I don't think I'd have the adrenalin left to work the hours I am used to just to set up my own quiet business. So for now I hold down the job I always dreamed of, and it holds me down too. We'll live with that truce for another few seasons!

TSF: Second Opinion

What the physio saw

Interesting fact for you. Just in case you ever become a footballer. Or the owner of a football club. Or, indeed, the administrator appointed by a football club when it hits the buffers.

I played for a club that went into administration. Previous owners and managers overspent and the squad that I was a part of paid for it. Not just by having their wages withheld, but through the pitchfork-wielding mobs that abused us on the pitch every Saturday and at the gates to the training ground every morning.

But we've covered this before. In short, it's not a nice place to be as a footballer.

Now then. An administrator becomes the legal owner of the business it has been brought in to salvage, and in order to perform a rescue operation they need to raise money to steady the books and do deals with the creditors.

Players are the obvious targets when performing a fire sale. They hold the most value but are also the biggest burden in terms of wages. Get them out. What next? Well, you'd be surprised.

On the first morning, a team of administrators turned up at

our training ground and made a beeline for the physio room. Medicine has excellent value and it is one of the first things the vultures go for at a well-stocked training ground. The medicine cabinet had padlocks on it to stop players taking whatever they wanted but the administrators had brought bolt cutters with them. They clipped each lock and the padlocks fell to the floor.

I looked at the physio, who was giving me an ankle strapping at the time. He gave me a smirk.

The administrators pulled the cupboards open.

Empty.

Who took all the medicine? It's a mystery. But I bet the physio saw.

POSTSCRIPT

A good physio stands apart from almost all the other people you encounter in football. Most become involved because they love the game: they love the buzz of the changing room, the routine, or the smell of the grass; they love the banter, the glory and the feeling that comes from knowing that they are doing something a huge number of people can only dream of doing; they like the superiority, the fame and the money.

Not physios. That's not what the game is about for them. Not many physios I know love football. They are concerned with the *people* who play football, not the sport itself. They are people of science who have medical curiosities to ponder and problems to solve, and that excites them. Physiological problems are presented to them as a result of sport, injuries that are not common in the outside world. It isn't the thought of watching Cristiano Ronaldo or Lionel Messi plying their trade from a heated seat in the dugout that keeps them coming back, it is the thought of what injury either player might sustain and how quickly the physio can get him back in action. That is the physio's match day, that is his ninety minutes, his personal war of attrition, and the glory is all his when he pulls it off. They walk through the door in the morning and have no idea what might be coming their way once training stops. Everybody else's job is, to an extent, chipped in granite. It's the same as it was yesterday, and tomorrow will be the same too.

Physios are medical staff, of course, but they are mates too. Almost all of the physios who treated me throughout my career routinely call to see how I am, and they do the same for my former team-mates. They understand that their care doesn't end just because our body is no longer up to the rigours of football – and they are also acutely aware of the degenerating mental state of former professional footballers.

Once a physio, always a physio. A physio can start a career in football as soon as he has the qualifications, and he can retire at sixty-five. I was closer to twenty-nine than I was to forty when I retired from football, and sure I can go back in as a coach or a scout, I could work my way up to become a manager, I could even buy a football club and have total control – if I could pull off a coup d'état in a wealthy nation. But it would never be the same. I'll never be a football player ever again. And that's where the problems begin for so many ex-footballers.

About six weeks after I retired from football, I began experiencing shortage of breath, cold sweats and a racing heartbeat every morning when I woke up. It became worse in a short space of time and was eventually diagnosed as anxiety attacks. They were brought on by the panic my body felt from falling out of its routine; the sheer terror I felt from thinking that I may have woken up late and missed the start of training or, worse, the kick-off to a match, was causing my body to go into shock. Pathetic isn't it? It doesn't take long for your body to fall to shit after leaving this game of ours, and it takes even less time for the brain to do the same.

I've since spoken to a few of my former team-mates who retired at a similar time to me. They too have been suffering with panic or anxiety attacks. It turns out it is as common as fuck among us. Twenty years ago ex-footballers would not be admitting such things to each other. But today we wear moisturizer and talk about our feelings, which is good news. Nobody said that progress was pretty – just smooth and buff.

It was depression that curtailed my drive to get fit again. Over a year has elapsed between me writing the introduction to this book and me writing the words you're reading now. But that's not to say that life hasn't been going on. Of course it has.

One night, recently, I put my kids to bed and set the house alarm. Every night the downstairs is set to kill anybody who attempts to break in and steal the stuff we used to own. In the ten years we've had it, the alarm has never been triggered. Never.

I brush my teeth and slip into bed. My wife asks me if I've set the alarm. I decide that I'm not even going to answer her this time. Every night for the last ten years she has asked me the same question.

'Have you put the bloody alarm on?' she shouts.

'For fuck's sake, yes!' I shout back.

We remain madly in love.

At 4.13 a.m. the house alarm goes off.

It's like an air raid siren. The kids scream in their beds. My wife screams. It's scary. We're either being robbed or are going to be hacked to death, it's difficult to tell in the dark.

I leap from the bed. Actually, 'leaping' does not do justice to my reaction. It's more akin to a bullet from a gun. Only faster obviously. People always used to say that my first two yards were quick, that the other ninety-eight were my problem. And true to form, just as I get into something resembling a stride, I feel something explode in the back of my leg. I've been shot. No, stabbed. My hamstring feels as if it has been sheared from the back of my leg. It is fucking painful but I refuse to scream. In this house, only kids and wives scream. In the following seconds I realize that I have sprung from my mattress so quickly that I have pulled my hamstring. Years of experience tell me that it's a grade three tear.

God, my bloody hamstring. Every time the muscle stretches it's like somebody wiggling a hunter's knife in the back of my leg.

The display panel on the wall tells me where entry has been forced. It reads: 'Kitchen'.

'Be careful,' says Mrs TSF as I tread on the first step down towards the kitchen and certain death. It's hard to tell if she's being genuine. It'll be difficult to be careful if somebody blows me away from ten yards with a shotgun.

I reach the ground floor (wankers have ground floors) and I poke my head around the corner into the kitchen. I see nothing and I hear nothing. The alarm sensors are flashing in every corner of the room, high above the floor where the corners of the room meet the ceiling. There are four of them because it's a rectangular room. Duh.

First, I check the back door. It's locked. The sensors must be playing up.

I check the first one and it seems OK. Then the second, and then the third. Nothing out of the ordinary here. I turn to look at the fourth, and while my bleary vision cannot determine why it looks different, my eyes have taken in enough photons to tell my brain that something about the image doesn't look quite right. I walk cautiously towards it and stop. Sitting on top of the sensor, steadily devouring a huge moth – most likely from my wallet – is the biggest spider I have ever seen. It has positioned itself directly over the sensor and it appears to be laughing at me between mouthfuls.

I fetch the vacuum cleaner. It's the tried and tested method for removing spiders in the TSF household. I'm angry. I have pulled my hamstring for an arachnid. How would he like it? Well it's all right for him, he can get by on the other seven legs. I was thinking of doing a 20K run tomorrow. OK I wasn't, but the spider didn't know that did he? Why would he? He's busy getting on with his life, eating moths and caring little for the blood pressure and heart murmurs of ex-footballers.

My anger subsides and gives way to a deep sense of worthlessness. I remember that I've been retired for a few years and I don't have training tomorrow so it's of little consequence that I have a hamstring injury, which would mean I couldn't train for six to eight weeks. I don't have a big game to get ready for on Saturday. I don't have a team that's relying on me. I don't have a place on the team sheet to keep. I don't have a manager to appease. I don't have to keep up an image for the TV or the newspapers. I don't have a pre-match interview to give. I don't have an appearance fee to win or a wage to earn. I don't have three points to celebrate or the feeling of camaraderie to look forward to. Tomorrow there will be no banter, no stories, no togetherness.

In the morning I call the only person in my phone book who can help me and, as expected, he answers.

'What have you done now?' he asks. Physios know their players, and they also seem to sense the urgency of their ringtone too.

'Hamstring,' I say.

'Right, let me finish up with this bunch of prima donnas and I'll drop in next week. How did you do it by the way?'

'Catching a spider,' I say.

'Ah yeah, of course. Just thinking out loud, given that your knees are shot to bits, wouldn't it be a good idea to get a bloody bike? You can still cycle with a pulled hamstring. Start working it now, it'll help.'

Bloody physios. They're always right when it comes to physiology. It's sickening.

Fortunately, Mrs TSF picks up on the subtle hints I drop that a bike would be a nice surprise for Christmas, which was at that point upon us. So here I am, helping myself. Hitting the road on a pretty nice-looking bike, knees feeling good, and with plans for veganism and a dry January firmly in place.

I get out there and feel truly exhilarated. I have not felt this kind of a burn in my legs since pre-season at my last Premier League club. I feel a small sense of purpose once more. The wind, the surroundings, the adrenalin. I even remember to stick out my arm when turning right. I don't know why all these cyclists have a problem with other traffic on the road: everybody is perfectly pleasant as they manoeuvre past while I notch up a steady average speed of 6kph. (Lance who?)

I approach the junction to my house. Behind me a Honda Civic brakes as I stick out my right arm – he could have overtaken me a while back but he is respectful. He clearly appreciates that I have just received this bike for Christmas and that, as an ex-footballer (recognizable even under a black helmet with questionable attire hugging my special places), I am helping myself. He respects the fact that it hasn't been an easy transition for me into civilian life, both mentally and physically. It's a lovely way to start the new year and reinforces my belief that people are fundamentally good. Even in dreary January.

'Speed up you fucking c**t!'

I couldn't see her, she was going too fast, but I heard her, and so did the family of five standing at the bus stop on the opposite side of the road.

I silently pray to any God that has ever been made up by any civilization that I hear a loud smash somewhere in the distance. It doesn't come. Bloody religion. Either God is out on his bike today or he drives a Honda Civic. Nonetheless, a miracle happens: I make it home. That in itself is enough to overshadow the incident.

When I return, the physio is waiting on my drive in his car. It's no Honda Civic. It is a car that suggests last season's Champions League bonus means that the local Mercedes garage won't have to open for the rest of the financial year.

Five minutes after the physio walks into my house and begins to look at my injured hamstring, and from his subsequent questions, I know that he has spotted the telltale signs that depression has crept up on me.

I have struggled with the divorce from professional football but I have at least tried to plug the gaps. I write books and I've got a couple of successful businesses and a loving family – at least I think they love me: Mrs TSF did seem to send me down those stairs when the house alarm went off fairly readily. But on this occasion I am exhibiting signs of depression and the physio reminds me of what I need to do to combat it. It's the slap round the face that I need, and it keeps me on the straight and narrow. But there are thousands of former footballers around the world who cannot do the same.

Last year the former Bordeaux and Norwich City player Cédric Anselin was ready to kill himself. He'd tried to end his life four years earlier but his wife had stopped him. Now aged forty, and living alone, Anselin couldn't see another way out.

As a player he was a precocious talent and represented the French Under-21 side. In 1996 Bordeaux were a European force having won the Ligue 1 title and contested the UEFA Cup final against Bayern Munich. They would lose 5-1 over two legs but Anselin was just nineteen years old and part of a team that included future World Cup winners Christophe Dugarry, Bixente Lizarazu and the great Zinedine Zidane.

Years later, feeling alone, abandoned and helpless, Anselin made one last desperate phone call. 'In the darkness, this light was shining from my phone and drew my attention,' he remembers. 'In a split second, I realized I needed to speak to someone, anyone.'

And do you know who Anselin called? He called Clarke

Carlisle, a former team-mate of Anselin's at Norwich City and another ex-player who had also tried to kill himself.

Everybody knows that footballers need to be babysat. Every manager will tell you that, every kitman, every physio, every other player even. Yet for some reason that logic is tossed aside when the player is no longer in sight, when he is sat at home with nothing but his thoughts, long after the circus has left town.

When you become a professional footballer, you become a member of the PFA for life. Yet no one from the PFA has ever contacted me to see how my transition has been since I retired from professional football. Nobody from the FA has called by, or dropped an email, or sent a text. Nobody from UEFA has bothered to send a carrier pigeon or a fax. And nobody from FIFA has ever apparently wondered, 'Whatever became of that old TSF fella?' Although in fairness most of them are busy in The Hague at the moment.

An exit interview upon retirement (or stepping out of the game) is something that football needs. It is embarrassing that it doesn't exist. The mental health issues of the ex-footballing community will become an epidemic in the next five years if we don't monitor players when they stop playing and instead leave it up to them to help themselves. You might say, 'Tough shit, fuck them, they've had all the money and the glory and the fame.' True. But that doesn't mean the problem doesn't exist.

I'm not ashamed to cry out. I'm not ashamed to be the person that calls it as it is. An anonymous person isn't beyond help either.

I'm asking the FA and the PFA for help. I'm asking you to help us all. Help us, please.